I WANT TO BE
A SEAL TEAM MEMBER,

I WANT TO SWIM
THE DEEP BLUE SEA.

I WANT TO LIVE
A LIFE OF DANGER,

PICK UP YOUR SWIM FINS
AND RUN WITH ME!

TRADITIONAL NAVY SEAL RUNNING CADENCE

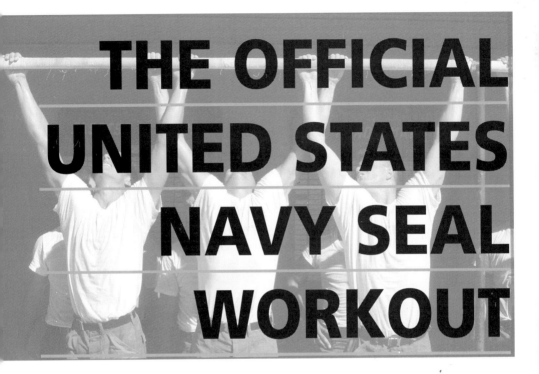

THE OFFICIAL UNITED STATES NAVY SEAL WORKOUT

RESEARCHED BY
ANDREW FLACH

PHOTOGRAPHED BY
PETER FIELD PECK

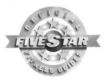

FIVE STAR PUBLISHING
NEW YORK

Five Star Publishing
An Independent Imprint of Hatherleigh Press

Five Star Publishing
1114 First Avenue, Suite 500
New York, NY 10021
1-800-906-1234
www.getfitnow.com

The use of the words Navy SEALs does not imply nor infer an endorsement,
either explicit or implicit, by the United States Navy or the Navy SEALs.

Before beginning any strenuous exercise program consult your physician. The
author and publisher of this book and workout disclaim any liability,
personal or professional, resulting from the misapplication of any of the
training procedures described in this publication.

A portion of the proceeds from the sale of each book will be donated to the
UDT-SEAL Museum Association and the UDT-SEAL Association.

All Five Star Publishing titles are available for bulk purchase, special
promotions, and premiums. For more information, please contact the manager
of our Special Sales Department at 1-800-906-1234.

Library of Congress Cataloging-in-Publication Data
Flach, Andrew, 1961 -
The official United States Navy SEAL workout / researched by
Andrew Flach ; photography by Peter Field Peck.
    p.   cm. — (The official Five Star fitness guides)
Includes bibliographical references   (p.).
ISBN 1-57826-009-4 (alk. paper)
    1. Exercise. 2. Physical fitness.
3. United States. Navy. SEALs. I. Peck, Peter Field, 1966 -   . II. Title. III. Series:
    Flach, Andrew, 1961 -   Official Five Star Fitness guides.
GV481.F553 1998   98-10159
613.7'1—dc21   CIP

Cover design by Gary Szczecina
Text design and composition by DC Designs
Photographed by Peter Field Peck
with Canon® cameras and lenses on Fuji® print and slide film
except photographs as noted: pages 11, 15, 16, 17, 21, 22 (bottom), 24, 56, 118

Printed on acid-free paper
10 9 8 7 6 5 4 3

YOU MAY *THINK* YOU'RE PHYSICALLY FIT NOW. BUT CAN YOU:

1. Swim 500 yards using breast and/or sidestroke in 12 minutes and 30 seconds, rest for 10 minutes, then
2. Do 42 pushups in two minutes, rest for two minutes, then
3. Do 50 situps in two minutes, rest for two minutes, then
4. Do eight pull-ups, rest for 10 minutes, then
5. Run 1.5 miles wearing boots and pants in 11 minutes and 30 seconds?

If you can, consider this: Those are just the requirements to get into Navy SEAL training—*before* the actual training begins! If you can't do the above, you'll be able to—no sweat—by the time you master the workout program described in this book. That's because the Navy SEAL workout is part of the actual SEAL training regime. Whether you want to be a SEAL or just be as physically fit as the most extensively trained combat force in the world, this program can help you achieve your goal.

ACKNOWLEDGMENTS

Thanks to the staff of the offices listed below for their contributions, which helped to make this book possible.

Navy Office of Information
Pentagon, Washington, DC

Special thanks to:
RADM Kendell Pease
Chief of Information

LT Wendy Snyder
Public Affairs Officer

Naval Special Warfare Center
Coronado, CA

Special thanks to:
RADM Thomas Richards
Commanding Officer

LCDR James Fallin
Public Affairs Officer

BM2 Kevin Blake
BUD/S Instructor

Our editorial team: Heather Ogilvie and Susan Ruszala
Our design and production team:
Dede Cummings, Matt Sharff, and Gary Szczecina.
Our logistics and support team: Kevin Moran and Bruce Slagle.
And to the many others who contributed to the
success of this mission:
Thank you!

DEDICATION

To the gallant Frogmen
and SEALs, past and
present. You are our
nation's finest. You have
served heroically. May
this book inspire others
to follow you to glory!

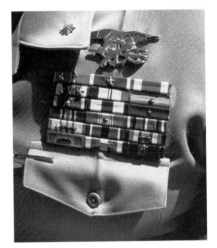

CONTENTS

ABOUT THE SERIES

The Official Five Star Fitness Guides are designed to provide a fresh new perspective on the subject of personal health and fitness by documenting the physical training regimens of the United States Armed Forces.

To bring you this exciting information, we have shouldered our gear in the hot midday sun, on cold frosty mornings, in the dark of night. No workouts and training schedules were reorganized to meet our needs. Nor did we ask. We wanted to bring to you what's REAL. I like to think of these books as "fitness documentaries"—because that's what they are!

We have talked extensively with many individuals responsible for the physical fitness and welfare of the men and women of America's Armed Forces. We have discovered the most powerful workout and physical training routines in the world. We bring them to you with the hope that you will be inspired to value your health and pursue fitness activities throughout your life.

Wherever possible, primary source material is utilized. Documentation, interviews, briefs—all were assembled and culled for details and insights.

One important note: These books are not designed to be follow-to-the-letter workouts. That was never our intention. These books are a collection of information on the subject of fitness and physical training in the US military, full of techniques, routines, hints, suggestions and tips you can learn from. Your workout should be individualized. We highly recommend you review your fitness plan with a certified trainer, coach, or other individual who possesses the proper knowledge to advise you in such a manner. And of course, consult your physician before commencing any new fitness program or before you intensify your current regimen.

Good luck and may lifelong fitness be your goal!

Andrew Flach
Peter Field Peck
January 1998

INTRODUCTION

How does one best describe the experience of witnessing Navy SEAL physical training? Do you write about the hot Southern California sun, the cloudless blue sky, the pounding surf ? Do you speak of the nonstop continuous training, the buzz of activity, the community of fitness? The seemingly countless pushups, pull-ups, situps, runs, and swims that each BUD/S student must perform if he is to become a Navy SEAL? Or do you speak of the men?

Quite honestly, the men I met that day at the Naval Special Warfare Center were a breed apart. The officers and instructors were exceptionally courteous. They were extremely knowledgeable and were eager to share their fitness information with me.

We met two BUD/S students when we needed to photograph the Navy SEAL Obstacle Course in action. They were among the most fit individuals I have seen. They ran the course flawlessly while Peter Peck photographed them tackling each obstacle. Many times Peter had to ask them repeat the obstacle so he could get a better camera angle to show important details. They obliged willingly, effortlessly. These two men were shining examples of America's youth: motivated, friendly, self-disciplined. Real role models.

When we arrived at the Naval Special Warfare Center the morning of our visit, August 18th, 1997, we were greeted by LCDR James Fallin, Public Affairs Officer. Commander Fallin advised Peter and me: "Be safe, have fun, and most importantly, tell the truth." I believe you'll find we accomplished all of those objectives, sir.

Enjoy this rare visit with our nation's elite US Navy SEALs.

Andrew Flach

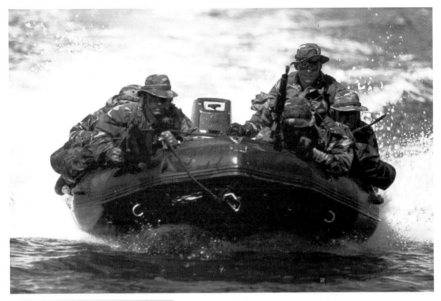

WHO ARE THE NAVY SEALS?

The SEALs are highly trained specialists that number less than one percent of the entire Navy. They are among the most elite fighting forces in the world, carrying out specialized missions that no other military unit can perform. The SEALs are extensively organized, trained, and equipped to conduct special operations, unconventional warfare, foreign internal defense, and clandestine operations in maritime and riverine environments. They are deployed worldwide, at a moment's notice, to support fleet and national operations. SEAL and SEAL Delivery Vehicle (SDV) Teams and Special Boat Units constitute the elite combat units of Naval Special Warfare. The extensive range of services and the outstanding combat record earn Naval Special Warfare a highly respected and revered reputation.

HISTORY OF THE SEALS

The history of the SEAL Teams dates back to 1943 when the first group of volunteers cleared obstacles from beaches chosen for amphibious landings during World War II. Though not yet known formally as SEALs, the volunteers in this mission constituted the first formal training of the Naval Combat Demolition Units (NC-DUs). The NCDUs earned a distinguished reputation at Utah and Omaha beaches in Normandy and in Southern France and throughout the Pacific.

After World War II, the Navy organized its first underwater offensive strike teams and the NCDUs were consolidated into Underwater Demolition Teams (UDTs). UDTs were deployed to Korea, where beginning in 1950 they saw combat at Inchon, Wonsan, Iwon, and Chinnampo and used guerrilla warfare. The UDT's missions included demolition raids on bridges and tunnels accessible from the water. In addition, they also conducted limited minesweeping operations in harbors and rivers.

UNCONVENTIONAL FIGHTERS

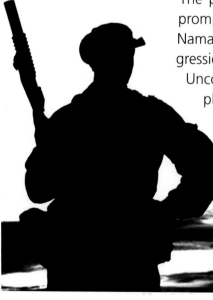

The perilous political climate of the 1960s prompted Secretary of Defense Robert McNamara to call for new ideas on counter-aggression. Later recommendations by the Unconventional Activities Committee emphasized use of assault landing, reconnaissance, patrolling, transport of troops and supplies, fire support, air support, and the infiltration and exfiltration of personnel. In addition, the committee recommended the increased study of mine warfare and guerrilla warfare functions. The proposal noted the formation of SEAL Teams, an acronym of sea, air and land teams, having a universal and extensive training in guerrilla warfare. SEAL units were further defined as having a specialized capability for special operations in rivers, bays, harbors, canals, and estuaries. The missions of these units were either overt or covert and the units were to attack enemy shipping and land men and matèriel on hostile shores.

In 1962, the first SEAL teams were commissioned to conduct unconventional warfare, counter-guerrilla warfare, and clandestine operations in both blue- and brown-water envi-

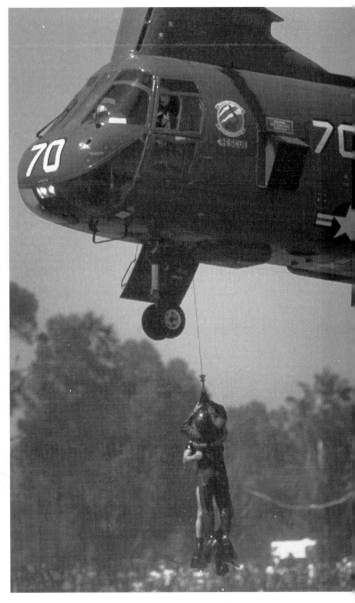

ronments. The Navy used former UDT forces to form these teams. The two teams formed were SEAL Team ONE on the West Coast and SEAL Team TWO on the East Coast. From 1962 to 1963, the Navy began to refine the basic structure for counterinsurgency warfare. The SEALs, along with other specialized units, became

17

PRE-BUD/S SCHOOLS

If you are interested in becoming a SEAL, the Naval Special Warfare BUD/S selection course provides an overview of SEAL Training and the Naval Special Warfare Community. The five-day course is offered to all active-duty Navy enlisted personnel from the Fleet, Service Schools, and Boot Camp. It is held at the Naval Training Command, Great Lakes. Applicants are temporarily assigned from their parent command to the selection course. The requirements for the course are the same as for BUD/S training. For further information, contact the Physical Training Rehabilitation Remediation office at (619) 437-0861 (DSN 577-0861).

the core of these highly specialized teams throughout the Vietnam War, where they compiled a successful record of combat missions.

THE SEALS TODAY

The changing face of world politics has created an even larger demand for the expansion of the SEAL teams since the close of the Vietnam War. The SEALs have recently conducted missions in Bosnia, Liberia, and the Persian Gulf. The SEALs have expanded in both size and capability, using former UDTs that have been redesignated as SEAL or SEAL Delivery Vehicle (SDV) Teams. Although the newly designated SEAL Teams acquired the SEAL mission, they retained the amphibious support mission inherited from the roots of the UDTs.

Today the SEALs are one of the country's most decorated combat units. Collectively, they have earned three Medals of Honor, numerous Navy Crosses, Legions of Merit, and Silver Stars, among hundreds of other medals.

SO YOU WANT TO BE A SEAL?

Many experts consider Navy SEAL training to be the toughest military training in the world. It's a challenging program that pushes men to their physical and mental limits. Here's how it begins.

The intense training is a continual process that begins at BUD/S (Basic Underwater Demolition/SEAL) in Coronado, California. BUD/S requires each participant to be self-motivated and physically fit. In addition to the physical training to improve stamina and strength, BUD/S tests your leadership ability as well. There is no room for substandard performance—at BUD/S your personal best is required every minute of every day. A regimented diet, exercise, and positive attitude are essential for success and a rewarding experience. The workouts in this book will help prepare you for the physical stress of the extremely thorough training program at BUD/S.

There are three Phases of training at BUD/S, described below.

FIRST PHASE: BASIC CONDITIONING.

First Phase consists of basic conditioning. The duration of First

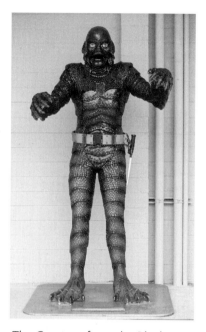

The Creature from the Black Lagoon, a gift from BUD/S Class 62, is located in the central courtyard of the BUD/S training center.

Phase is eight weeks. The physical conditioning consists of running, swimming, and calisthenics, and grows more difficult as the weeks progress. Students are required to participate in weekly four-mile timed runs in boots, timed obstacle courses, and swim distances up to two miles wearing fins in the ocean. They also learn small boat seamanship.

The fifth week of First Phase is called "Hell Week." During Hell Week, there are five and a half days of continuous training with a maximum of four hours of sleep. This week is designed to test the individual's physical and mental motivation while still in First Phase and relies heavily on teamwork. The last three weeks of First Phase teach methods of conducting hydrographic surveys and how to prepare a hydrographic chart.

SECOND PHASE: DIVING.

The successful completion of First Phase proves that you are ready for more serious training. Second Phase concentrates on combat Self Contained Underwater Breathing Apparatus (SCUBA). The diving skills you learn during this seven-week period train you in the skills that separate SEALs from all other Special Operations forces. Although the physical training used in First Phase continues, students must complete the four-mile runs, two-mile swims, and obstacle course in less time. Students concentrate on two types of SCUBA: open circuit (compressed air) and closed circuit

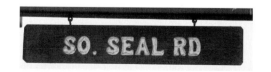

(100 percent oxygen). The ultimate goal is to train the student with basic combat swimmer skills to qualify as a combat diver. Again, a progressive dive schedule is used to emphasize the basic combat skills needed in order to qualify as a combat diver.

THIRD PHASE: LAND WARFARE.

This is a physically intense ten-week training phase with the focus on demolition, reconnaissance, weapons, and tactics. Students learn land navigation, small-unit tactics, rappelling, military land and underwater explosives, and weapons training. In addition, the run distances increase and the minimum passing times are once again lowered for the runs, swims, and obstacle course. Students apply techniques learned in the training program during the final four weeks on San Clemente Island in California.

After graduation from BUD/S, there is additional training. Before reporting to their first Naval Special Warfare Command, graduates receive three weeks of basic parachute training at the Army Airborne School, Fort Benning, Georgia. Navy corpsmen who

ARE YOU NAVY SEAL MATERIAL?

In addition to passing a physical screening test to enter the Navy's SEAL training (known as BUD/S), you must also meet these general requirements:

1. Pass a diving physical exam
2. Pass an eye exam—eyesight cannot be worse than 20/40 in one eye and 20/70 in the other eye and must be correctable to 20/20 with no color blindness
3. Minimum ASVAB score: VE + AR = 104, MC = 504.
4. Be 28 years old or younger
5. Be male

If you meet these requirements, start planning your Navy career today. Call your local Navy recruiter. Start the workout program immediately—with motivation, you can incorporate these exercises into a busy high school or college schedule.

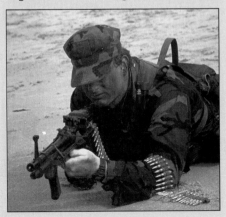

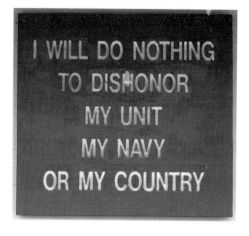

complete BUD/S and Basic Airborne Training also attend two weeks of Special Operations Technicians Training at the Naval Special Warfare Center, Colorado. In addition, they participate in a 30-week course of instruction in diving medicine and medical skills called 18-D (Special Operations Medical Sergeant Course). During this time, students receive training in burns, gunshot wounds, and trauma.

Qualified personnel are awarded a SEAL Naval Enlisted Classification (NEC) Code and Naval Special Warfare Insignia after the successful completion of a six-month probationary period with a Team. New combat swimmers serve the remainder of their first enlistment (two and a half to three years) in either a SEAL Delivery Vehicle (SDV) or SEAL Team. Upon re-enlistment, members may be ordered to additional training and another SDV or SEAL Command where they will complete the remainder of a five-year sea tour. Advanced courses include Sniper, Diving Supervisor, language training, and SEAL Tactical Communications. There are also shore duty opportunities available in research and development as well as instructor duty and overseas assignments.

For information about becoming a Navy SEAL, see the Recruitment Information in the back of the book.

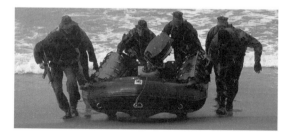

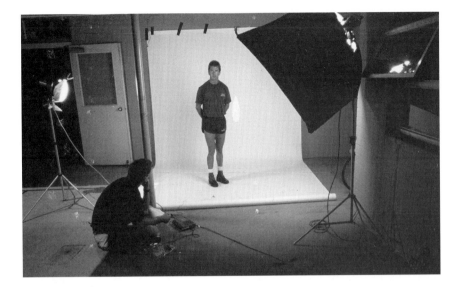

MEET BM2 KEVIN BLAKE,
NAVY SEAL INSTRUCTOR

We were fortunate to have an experienced BUD/S instructor, BM2 Kevin Blake, share his fitness knowledge with us during our visit to the Naval Special Warfare Center. Kevin demonstrated the stretching and PT exercises for us, as well as providing insight into SEAL training in all Phases of BUD/S.

Kevin has been a Navy SEAL for almost 15 years. Since 1982, he has been a member of SEAL Team 2, SEAL Team 3, and SEAL Team 5. As a Navy SEAL, Kevin has served in Europe, the Mediterranean, Southeast and Southwest Asia, and the Western Pacific. In addition, Kevin spent a year in Kodiak, Alaska, as a Winter Warfare Instructor. In his spare time, Kevin is an avid rock climber, cyclist, and triathlete.

Kevin is currently asssigned as Fourth Phase BUD/S instructor. Fourth Phase is a special pre-training Phase, and precedes First Phase. It is called Fourth Phase because it is the newest Phase of BUD/S to be developed. Fourth Phase concentrates heavily on physical conditioning and was designed to help BUD/S candidates ready themselves to enter First Phase.

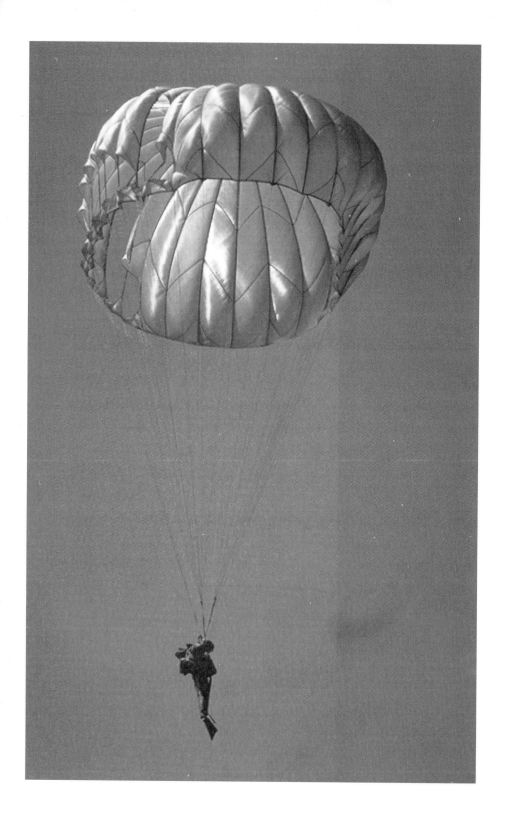

STAYING MOTIVATED

A BUD/S student's most valuable motivation comes from his brothers-in-training. The BUD/S class pulls together. Unique about SEAL training is the pressure and stress on the students — which they sometimes can perceive as a negative — but the students do have a positive source to tap into.

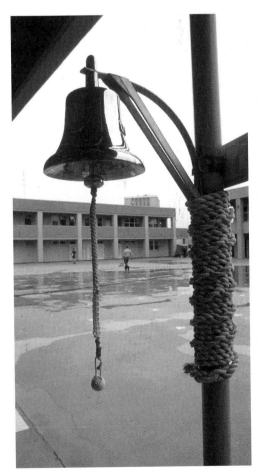

Tradition has it that if a BUD/S student decides to drop from training, he must ring The Bell three times and place his helmet on the ground beneath it. This gesture is repeated many times during a BUD/S class. The dropout rate can be as high as 75% or greater.

25

They develop spirit as a class of men going through something that's demanding, challenging, and desirable.

An infectious spirit develops within the class, especially as SEALs go through training and come closer to the end. They start to gel as a class—you can really see and feel the motivation.

But what if you're not a BUD/S student, and maybe you're interested in being a SEAL someday, thinking about going to BUD/S, and working out at home to get yourself in shape? What then? What can you do to stay motivated? Find somebody to be a support person—someone who shares your dreams and goals and values. You can help each other to stay motivated, and by training together you'll get awesome results!

Positive mental imagery is also important. Have a clear idea of your goal. Keep focused on that image. Keep thinking of it. Make it a positive mental image of who, what, and where you want to be and then go for it! Self-motivation is a powerful tool.

Here's one example to make your training more effective. Let's say you're running down the beach or road. Think of yourself as being in a race. Think of the road as being lined with people who are cheering for you. You'll notice your form getting better—you'll run faster, harder. Next thing you know you're done! You've had a great workout using positive mental imaging as a self-inspirational tool.

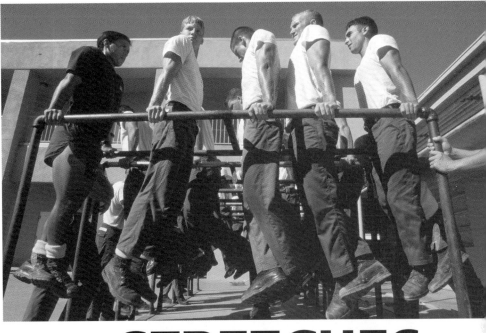

STRETCHES

INTRODUCTION

Stretching is often the warmup for exercise programs, but SEALs prefer to warm up *before* they start to stretch. If you go right into stretching cold, it's not only painful but it can be injurious too. You might want to take an easy run, say two or three miles and then stretch. At that point you will be warmed up and ready to go. Stretch—and *then* get into the workout. If you don't have the time to run first, try a 15-minute fast walk, do jumping jacks, or perform any other calisthenics that get the blood pumping.

HURDLER

Sitting on the floor,
form a 90° angle with your legs as shown. Relax. Feel the weight go down into your leg muscles and then gently lean forward without bouncing. A little bit of pulsing is okay just to increase that stretch. Reach out and grab the palm of your foot. Relax everything a little more and just pull into it—not so it causes pain, but it should feel good. You do not want to cause pain. Keep your back straight. Eventually lie down on the leg. It takes a while—weeks and months of stretching—before you attain maximum flexibility.

The second part of the Hurdler Stretch is to lie back and stretch out as in the second photo. It's important to let your body go into a natural position, where everything is relaxed and you can concentrate on the muscle that needs to be stretched. Hold for 30 seconds, then lean over.

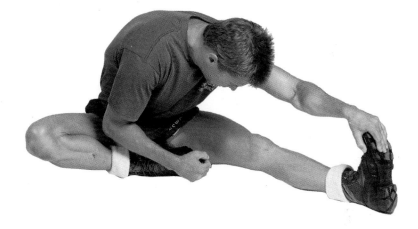

MODIFIED HURDLER

In the Modified Hurdler, bring your foot in as the photo shows. This stretch is easier on the back than the regular Hurdler, and it also helps stretch out the lower back. It's just as much of a lower back stretch as it is a hamstring stretch. Stretching out the lower back is important and becomes even more important as a person ages.

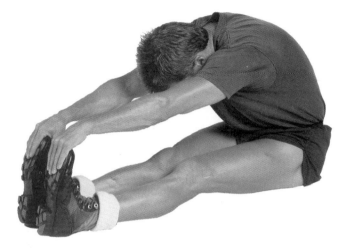

SITTING HEAD TO KNEE

The Sitting Head to Knee is a double hamstring stretch. Put both legs straight out. Grab the toes. This is another full back-of-the-leg stretch, from the calves to the buttocks. Hold and pull down gradually—not causing pain—and you might want to rock gently from side to side a little bit just to feel the stretch go around the sides of your legs.

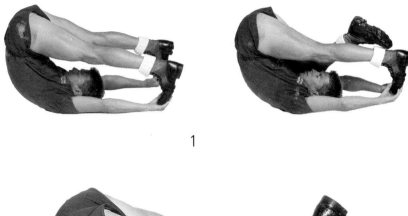

1   2

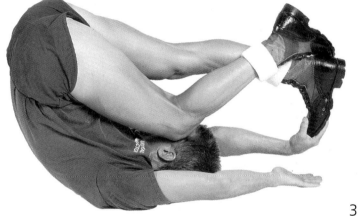

3

BACK ROLLERS

The Back Roller is a really good back and hamstring stretch. Relax and just let gravity pull you down. Then you can let go with one leg and cock your hips so that the hip that's connected to the leg that's being stretched helps stretch the back muscles down the length of your spine. Repeat the stretch on the other side.

31

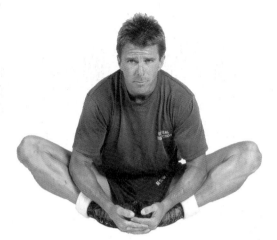

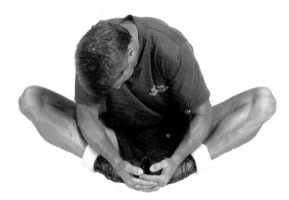

BUTTERFLY STRETCH

The Butterfly is a favorite. It's very relaxing. Just put both soles of your feet together and bring them in close. The point is to stretch the tendons and the ligaments in the groin. Get your feet in as close as you can, flat together, and then push down on your shins and calves with your elbows. Stretch with your neck and head down. You can also rock back and forth gently—nothing real drastic or jerky. This increases flexibility all the way around.

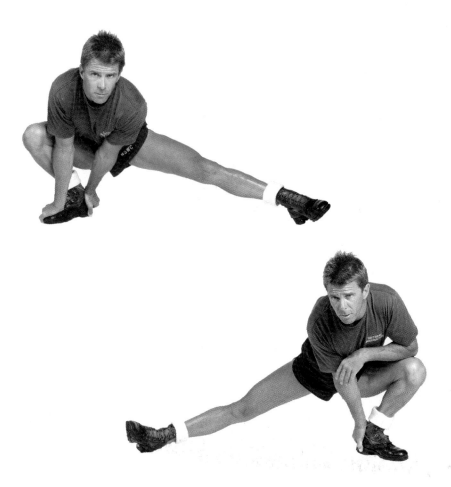

GROIN STRETCH

Stand with legs a little wider than shoulder length apart. The goal is to stretch your tendons from the inside of your thigh down to your knee. You might want to put a hand on your heel as shown. It provides support and it keeps your other leg down flat. Relax your body and lean into the stretch. Repeat on the other side.

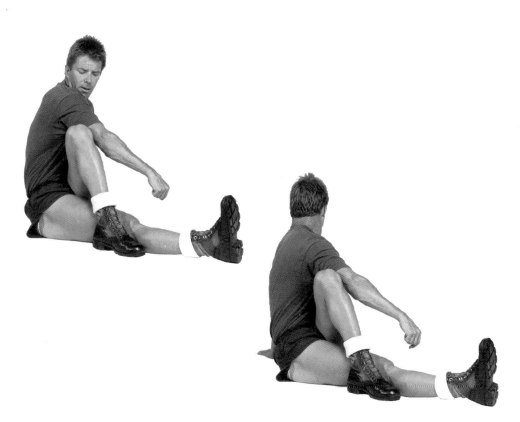

ILIO TIBIAL BAND STRETCH

To start, put your right leg out flat and cross your left leg over so that the outside of the heel is by the knee. The effective part of this stretch is putting your elbow on the outside of your crossed-over knee, pushing on it, and turning so you can feel the stretch all the way through the upper hamstrings, through the gluteal region, and into the lower back. Turn your head as you stretch. Repeat on the other side.

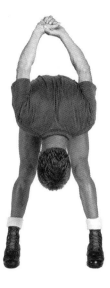

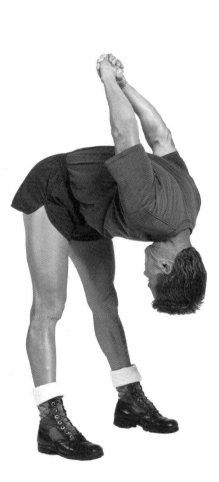

SWIMMER STRETCH

Bend over as shown, grabbing a wrist with one hand or interlocking your fingers, and then pull it back and gently stretch out the lats and the frontal deltoids. The Swimmer Stretch is something you might want to try with your workout buddy for maximum effectiveness, although it can be performed individually too.

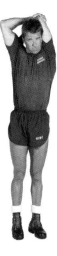

TRICEPS STRETCH

Put your right elbow up on the right side of the head, placing your right hand in the middle of your shoulder blades. Grab your right elbow with your other hand, and then pull it back, nice and easy, stretching your triceps. This can turn into a pretty good lat or side stretch if you bend to your left as shown. Reverse arm positions to stretch the other triceps and side.

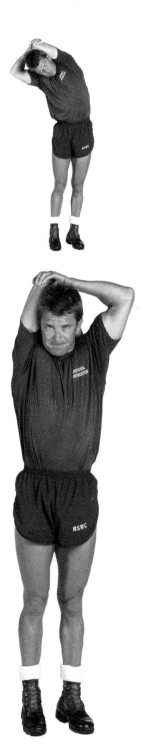

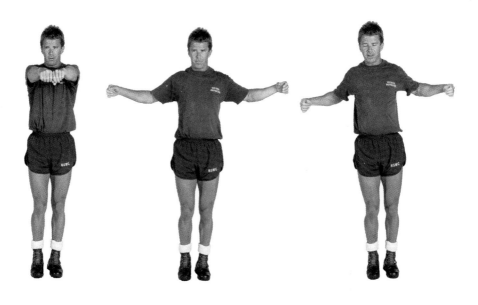

PRESS-PRESS-FLING

Press-Press-Fling starts out with your arms straight out front, horizontal. Then bring them back in a butter-fly-like chest movement with your elbows bent at a 90° angle—snap it back to get the most range of mo-tion. That's the Press. Do it twice. Press-Press. Be care-ful not to snap too hard. And avoid this stretch if you are recovering from a shoul-der injury. The Fling is ac-complished by opening your arms nice and wide and

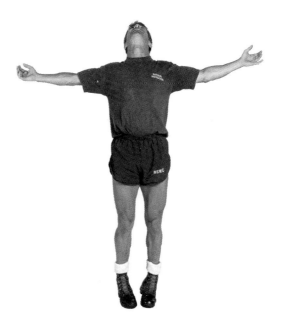

snapping back. At the same time, come up on your toes and arch your back. Press-Press-Fling. It's easier than it sounds.

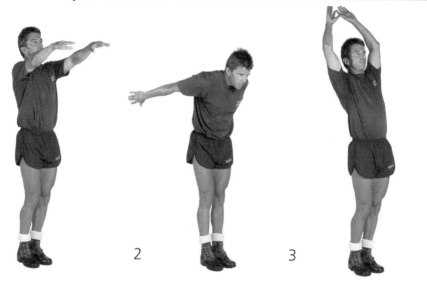

1   2   3

UP, BACK AND OVER

Up, Back and Over starts with both arms at your side. Lift your arms straight up. That's the Up. Then fling them behind you, like in the Swimmer's Stretch. That's the Back. Return to the starting position and then do a big reverse arm circle. Stretch it all the way around back to the starting position. That's the Over. Then repeat.

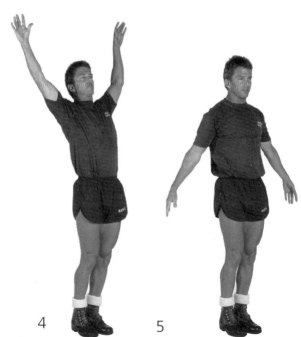

4   5

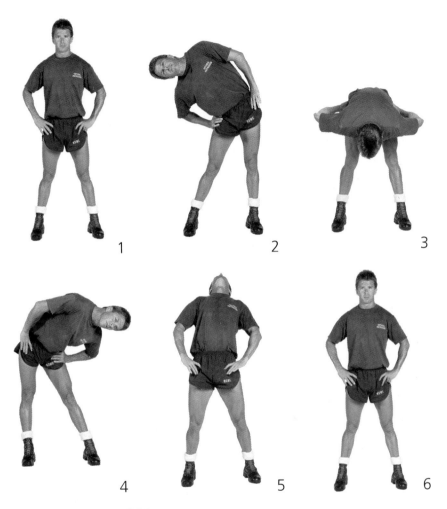

1

2

3

4

5

6

TRUNK ROTATION

Hands on your hips, feet about shoulder width apart. It should be a stable and comfortable stance. Starting off nice and slow, bend at your waist to the right side. Lean into it a bit. Return to the start position. Bend to the front. Return. Bend to the left. Return. Then bend to the back. And return. Half way through the desired number of repetitions, it is recommended that you reverse direction, starting to the left.

39

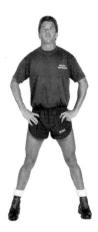

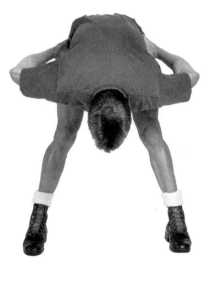

TRUNK BENDING FORE AND AFT

Trunk Bending Fore and Aft is pretty simple. Hands on your hips, feet about shoulder width apart. Bend to the Front. One. Return to the starting position. Two. Bend to the Rear. Three. Return. Four. As in all exercises, keep an even tempo as you count the repetitions. One, two, three, ONE. One, two, three, TWO. One, two, three, THREE. And so on. It keeps your mind clear so you can remember how many you've done. Or how many more you have to do!

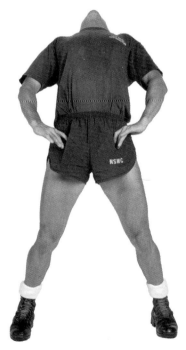

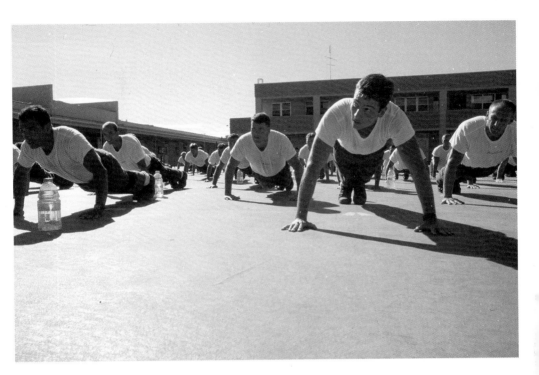

UPPER
BODY

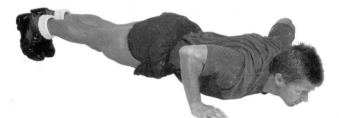

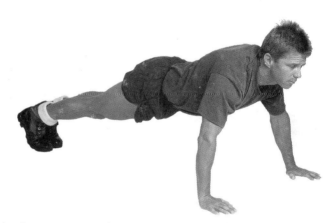

PUSHUPS

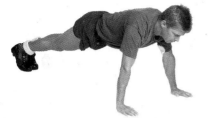

Everyone should be familiar with this standard physical training (PT) exercise. A Navy SEAL does many of these to get strong. Follow the instructions carefully and focus on developing proper technique and soon you'll be cranking out hundreds of pushups. Starting position is shown in the top photo. Hands are a comfortable width apart—a little wider than the shoulders is typical. Have your feet together and lower yourself down to the deck leaving less than a fist's width of room between your chest and the ground. Keep your back perfectly straight—the SEALs emphasize a completely straight body when performing this classic pushup or its variations. Don't let your back sag or your body bend at the waist with your buttocks higher than your back. Not only does it look bad, you can hurt yourself in the process. Learn them and do them right!

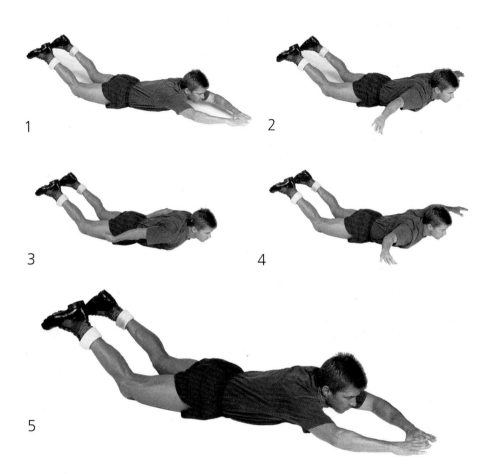

1
2
3
4
5

ARM HAULERS

These are good to add on at the end of the pushups series. Get down on your belly, feet and arms up off the deck so everything's arched, with your arms stretched out in front of the head. Following a full range of motion, sweep all the way back to the thighs and all the way forward again. Do it as a four-count exercise: one, two, three, ONE. One, two, three, TWO. One, two, three, THREE. The Arm Hauler is like a breaststroke on land. Keep it nice and slow—it's torture for the delts.

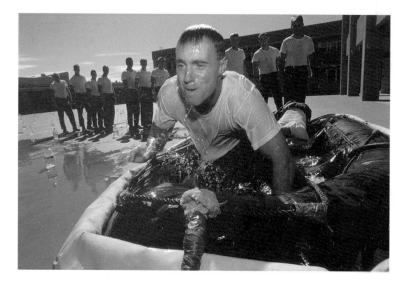

During Grinder PT sessions, SEAL candidates fill up one or two IBSs (INFLATABLE BOAT SMALL) with water. They do it for a couple of reasons. If a guy seems to be overheating they will send him to the IBS to cool off. They can even ask to do it if they want to—they can quickly douse themselves without having to run all the way out to the surf.

Sometimes, if a guy's not performing and needs a little motivation, the instructors send him to the IBS to help him reconsider his motivation. The water can get a little nasty after several dozen overheated BUD/S students go for a dunk. Take my word: Don't try this at home!

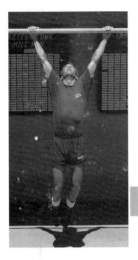

PULL-UPS
AND DIPS

What's the secret to the perfect pull-up?

Here are a few tips. Keep your back arched. Think of your arms as a set of hooks—try not to bring your biceps into play too much. Isolate your back. Pull-ups are a back movement, though your arms will inevitably get pumped. And don't forget to stretch.

Let's say you can do seven pull-ups, how are you going to do eight?

Here are two solid ways of cranking out more pull-ups: First, find a gym with a Lat Pull-Down machine and start adding weight up to 10 or 25 pounds more than your body weight and do five solid pull-downs. Then reduce the weight to 10 or 25 pounds below your body weight and go for eight or nine pull-downs. With this technique you're getting accustomed to doing more of the pull-up movement plus you're adding resistance. It will make you stronger to lift your own body weight when doing actual pull-ups.

A second way to increase your ability to perform proper Navy SEAL dead-hang pull-ups (and we mean this—no bicycling or kicking your legs to get up and over the bar) is to work out with a buddy. Your buddy can actually assist you by pushing upward on your hips or on your lower back as you do them, just enough to help you squeeze out a couple more on the pull-up bar.

Navy SEALs do many regular pull-ups and pull-up variations.

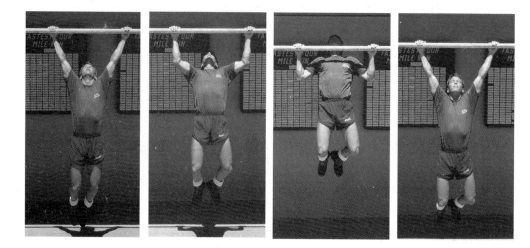

REGULAR GRIP

The regular grip pull-up is performed routinely. Grab the pull-up bar with your arms spaced a little wider than your shoulders. Keep your thumb and fingers on the same side of the bar. From a dead-hang, thinking of the arms as hooks, work your back, not your arms. Keep your back arched. Look up. Pull yourself up over the bar and lower yourself in a controlled fashion. Concentrate on utilizing proper technique for all of the pull-up variations. Form is key.

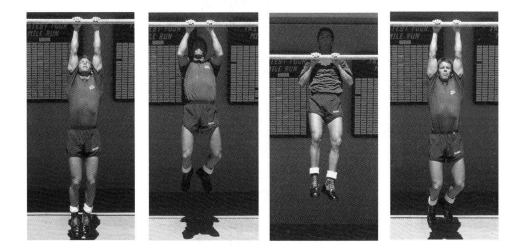

CLOSE GRIP

Grab the pull-up bar palms facing out, your hands a couple of inches apart. Same technique as in the regular grip pull-up. Back arched. Hands like hooks. Do them right. Notice in the photo the true dead-hang. There is absolutely no leg motion whatsoever. If you are having trouble keeping your legs still, or if you are on the tall side, you might want to bend your knees a bit and cross your legs at the ankles. This will increase your stability and will reduce the tendency to bicycle.

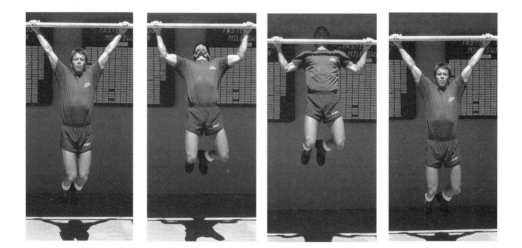

WIDE GRIP

Wide grip pull-ups are definitely challenging. Set your arms as wide as possible—but not so it's uncomfortable. The same technique applies: Hands like hooks. Use your back, and your deltoids get a great work-out. Pull yourself up and lower yourself down. Nice and easy. Always in control.

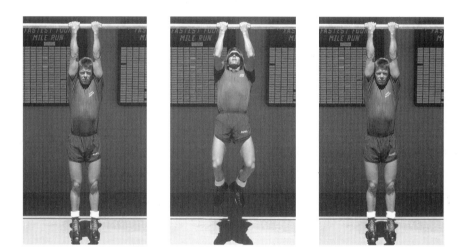

REVERSE GRIP

Otherwise known as the "chin-up" or "curls," reverse grip pull-ups are sometimes referred to as "curls for the girls." Not that they are easy, mind you. Especially after you have cranked out a total of 50 or 60 pull-up combinations in the hot sun.

Reverse grip pull-ups are performed exactly like the close-grip pull-ups, only you reverse your grip so your palms are facing toward you (again keeping fingers and thumbs on the same side of the bar). Set your hands a few inches apart and perform the exercise. You will find this pull-up variation uses more biceps strength than the others.

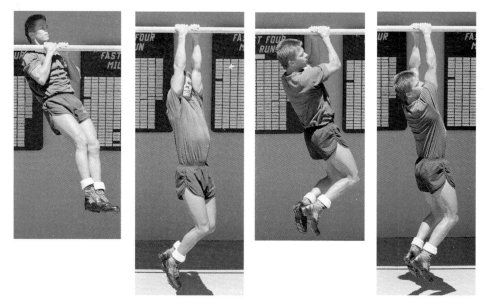

CLIFFHANGERS

The Cliffhanger is a challenging pull-up. It provides a multi-dimensional workout: biceps, delts, and lats all share in the fun. Start by standing directly underneath the pull-up bar and turn so your body is perpendicular to it. Grab the bar with your right hand and then grab the bar with your left hand, making certain that your left hand is furthest away from you. Make certain that both hands touch. Now pull yourself up, bringing your right shoulder to meet the bar, as shown in the photo. Lower yourself in a controlled manner. Do the exact same pull-up again. And again. When you are halfway through your set, switch your grip and do your Cliffhangers on the left side.

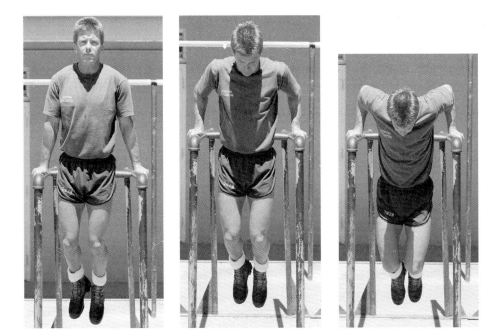

DIPS

Dips are another staple in Navy SEAL workouts. Proper form is essential. Your back should be kept straight and arched. Keep your elbows in. Thumbs facing forward. Lower yourself in a controlled manner until your elbows are just at a 90° angle. Don't bend further than 90°—it's an invitation for injury. Come up in smooth motion and avoid locking your elbows when at the starting position.

Workout Tip: If you want to work the chest more, look down and it will put more stress on the chest. If you want to work the triceps more, look up and you'll be working the triceps more.

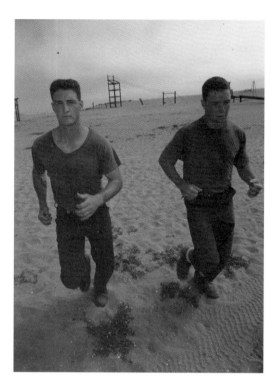

THE RUNNING PROGRAM

SEALs typically run three- to four-mile runs down the beach during training. Sometimes, depending on the tide and who's leading the run, they'll run down on the hard-packed sand at low tide or up on the soft sand, which makes for harder running. SEALs sprint on certain days. They also do "berm" runs: over the berm (which is like a sand dune), down to the water line, and turn around and run back over the berm again.

Long runs are great for building stamina. Sprints are essential for developing speed and strength.

"THE ONLY EASY DAY WAS YESTERDAY"

THE SWIMMING PROGRAM

Navy SEALs are water-borne warriors. Hence they do a lot of swimming. Their swims are varied to prepare them for combat mission swim conditions. Here's an example of a pool swim "evolution" designed to build strength and stamina.

The swim starts with a warmup of 800 to 1,000 meters using the "underwater recovery stroke" or SEAL combat swimmer stroke, which is a very aggressive form of the traditional sidestroke. After the

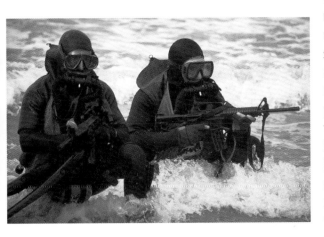

warmup they will do 50-meter swims on the minute, meaning a new swimmer departs every minute, and each swimmer is expected keep pace. It's a lot to expect for some people so the instructors inevitably break it into groups of slower and faster swimmers. The goal is to keep the 50 meters per minute pace.

They'll perform about ten of these relays and then go to 100m/1 min:20 sec. A swimmer will depart on a 100-meter swim every 1:20. This is performed for a specified number of repetitions, perhaps five or ten. Then they go to 200-meter relays—fewer repetitions, of course—with timed departures every 2:30. Just another easy day in the life of a Navy SEAL.

SEALs also routinely perform ocean swims, and learn drown-proofing techniques, underwater knot tying, open and closed circuit SCUBA, hydrographic reconnaissance, and other specialties depending upon the Phase of their training.

LOWER BODY

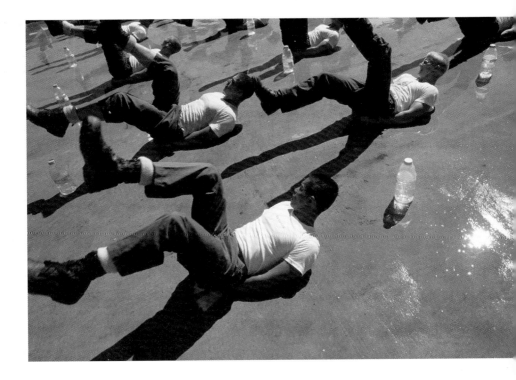

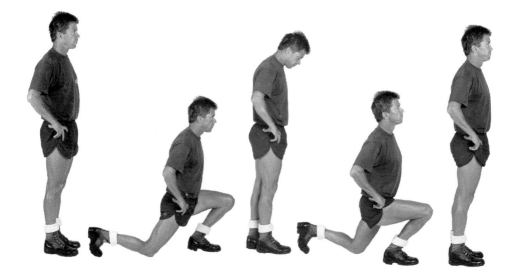

LUNGES

The importance of excellent leg strength to a Navy SEAL goes without saying. The first exercise is the Lunge. Start with your hands on your hips to get them out of the way. Some guys in the past have put their hands behind their head—this is not advisable as it pulls down on the neck, throwing you way out of form and risking injury. To perform a proper lunge keep your back straight and protected. This is not a down-up exercise. It is a step forward-down-up motion that is repeated again and again. Try these in reverse for fun (but look where you are going!).

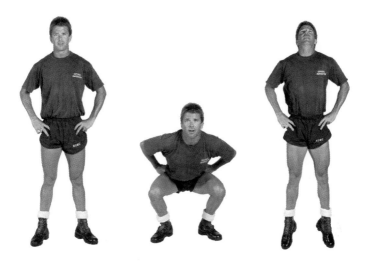

SQUAT LEAPS

A regular Squat is a down-up motion. What SEALs do to make it interesting is to turn it into a jump. This kind of explosive training is
known as plyometrics. Plyometric training is used in many sports,
such as basketball, where power and speed are required goals. Start
with your feet about shoulder width apart, toes pointed out so your
knees align properly to minimize injury risk. Now with your hands on
your hips, lower yourself so your knees are bent to about a 90° angle. Then from this position, propel yourself upward as if a C-4
charge went off under the soles of your feet. Land safely and repeat.

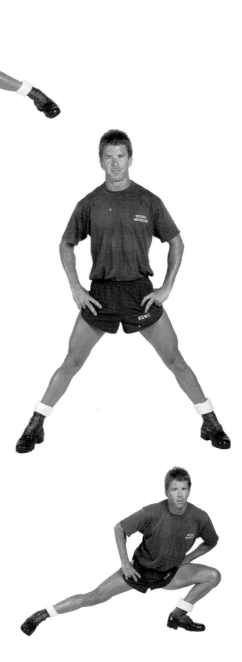

SIDE LUNGE

Although this looks like the Groin Stretch, it is performed differently. It's not a stretch, it's an exercise. Starting with your legs wider than shoulder width apart (as shown), lower yourself to the right by bending your right leg and shifting your weight to the right. Your knee should be just about 90°. Push up off your right foot and return to the start position. Now do the same on your left side. Repeat the exercise right-left-right-left.

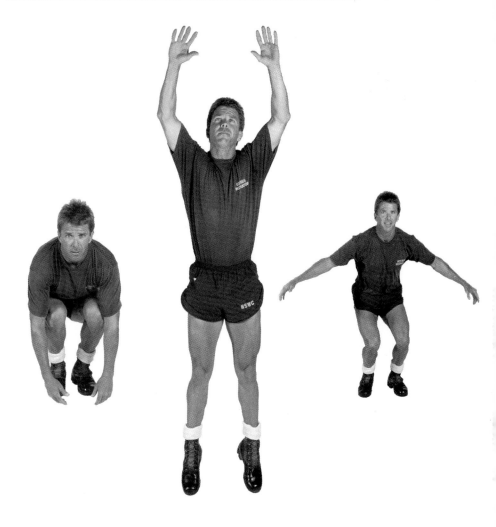

STAR JUMPERS

Another excellent plyometric.

Start in a squat position as shown. Now with a burst of energy, jump up with your hands high above your head. Grab a star while you're up there. After all, with the Navy SEALs *anything's* possible!

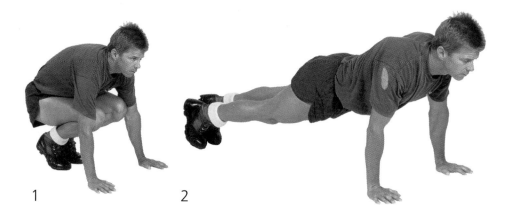

1   2

EIGHT-COUNT BODY BUILDER

The Eight-Count Body Builder is a Navy SEAL PT classic. It really is a unique exercise combining a variety of moves and muscles and the result is a powerful PT exercise that works the upper body, lower body, and cardiorespiratory system. Some might call it the mother of all pushups.

Here's how you do it. Begin in a standing position. Move to a squat position with your arms slightly more than shoulder width apart and count "1." Thrust your legs straight back, count "2." Keeping your back straight, lower yourself in a picture perfect pushup "3" and up "4." Kick your legs apart like a scissor "5" then kick them back together "6." Pull your legs back in a reverse thrust motion "7." And stand "8." You have just performed one Eight-Count Body Builder. Congratulations!

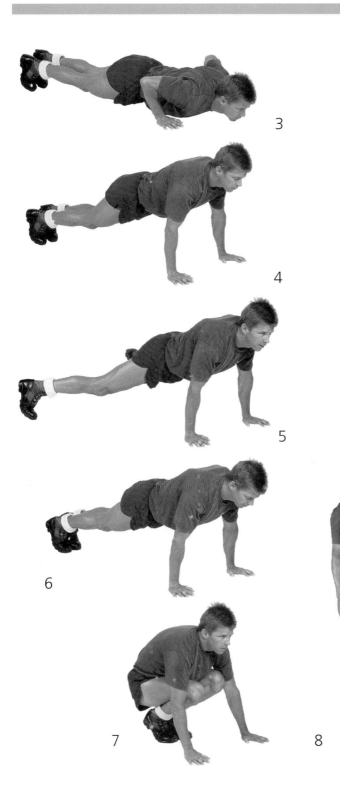

3

4

5

6

7

8

ABDOMINALS

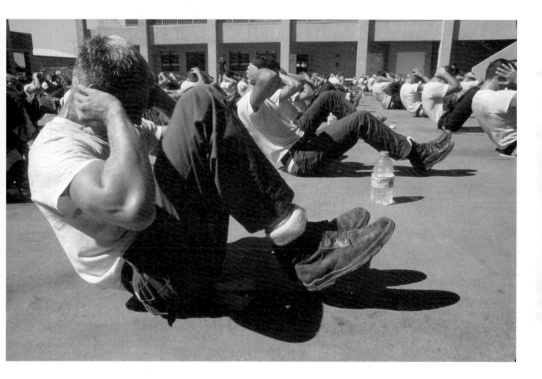

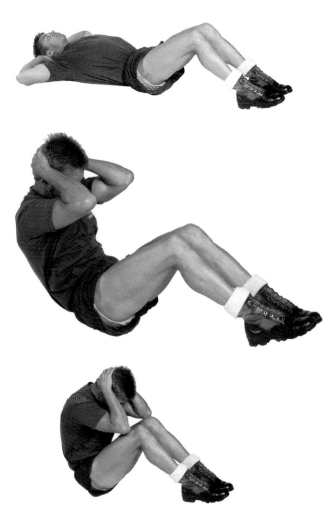

SITUPS

Another PT classic. Learn to do them right: start with knees bent, at a comfortable angle, hands clasped behind the head, elbows on the deck. Come up, touch your elbows to your thighs, and return. It's important to keep your back rounded. Guys who are not in good shape tend to arch the back—an injury invitation. So to reduce your risk, roll up and roll down, gently!

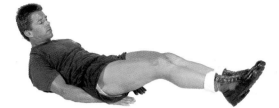

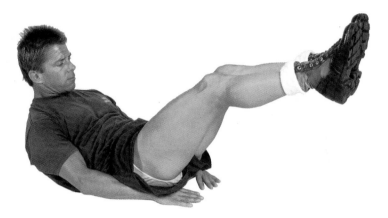

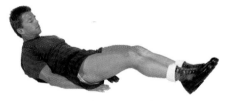

LEG LEVERS

Leg Levers are a lower abdominal exercise. To begin, take your hands and form a sort of "cradle" for your body (see photo). This arm position encourages the back to stay rounded —again to re-duce risk of injury or strain. With your back rounded on the ground, lift your feet about six inches off the ground. Don't lock your legs out straight; keep them a little flexed. Concentrate on using your lower abs and lift your legs from six inches up to maybe 26 or 30 inches, max. Repeat. Repeat. Repeat.

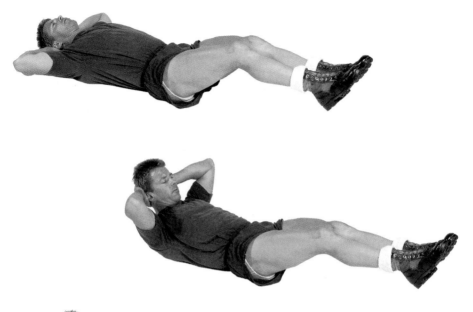

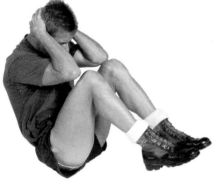

ATOMIC SITUPS

Welcome to the Nuclear Age! Why is it called an Atomic Situp? Well, after two cycles of 20 of these you'll feel like someone dropped an A-Bomb on your belly. Lie on your back and place your hands behind your head as shown. Extend your legs and lift your feet about six inches off the deck, keeping your legs slightly flexed. That's the starting position. Perform a situp while at the same time pulling your knees into your chest. It's a tough one, no doubt. Just keeping your balance is challenging.

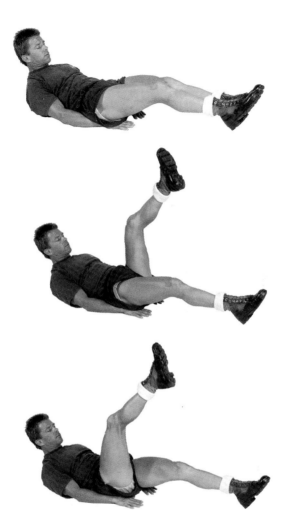

BACK FLUTTER KICKS

Navy SEALs do a lot of swimming. Back Flutter Kicks are a great way to strengthen your hip flexors—muscles used consistently during long ocean swims. Back Flutter Kicks are a traditional and staple PT exercise. SEALs do a lot of these. Starting position is the same as in Leg Levers. Start kicking. Keep your range of motion between six inches to 36 inches max. It's a four-count exercise. One, two, three, ONE. One, two, three, TWO. One, two, three, THREE. And so on.

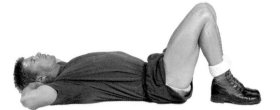

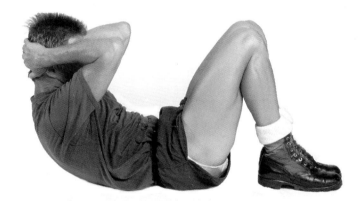

CRUNCHES — HEEL IN CLOSE

SEALs do Crunches with the heels in really close—as close as you can get them. Start with your hands behind your head as shown, knees bent and heels in tight, and using your abs, lift yourself to the crunch position. Do it slowly and with a controlled motion to get the most out of this crunch. Avoid pulling your head up with your hands! This is a sure way to strain your neck and cause injury.

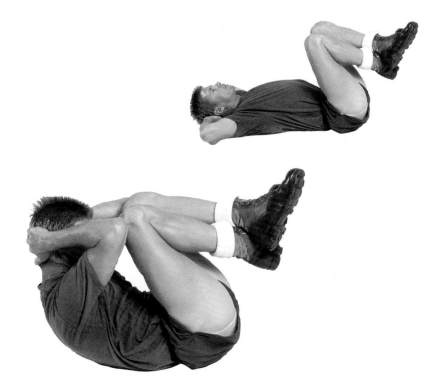

CRUNCHES — LEGS UP

The Legs Up Crunch is a traditional Navy SEAL ab exercise. A strong torso is a key to performing the many rigorous activities which are just a day's work for the SEALs. Doing Crunches will add to your overall ability to swim, run, climb ropes, and run the Obstacle Course, for example. Start with your hands behind your head as shown, legs up and knees bent at a 90° angle. Cross your ankles to create stability in your legs and lift yourself to the crunch position. Again, do it slowly and don't lift your head off the deck with your hands.

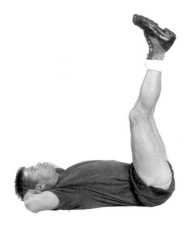

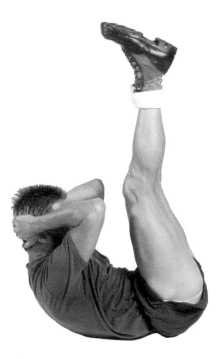

EXTENDED LEG CRUNCHES

The Extended Leg Crunches are another variation. By extending your legs vertically, as shown, creating a 90° angle at the hips, you are able to concentrate all your firepower on your ab muscles. Keeping your legs in the air adds to the intensity of the crunch. Do these slowly and hold the crunch position for a two count if you desire a greater challenge.

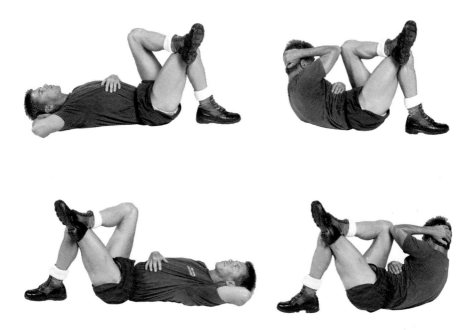

CROSS-LEGS SITUPS

This is designed as a Side Crunch for the intercostals, obliques, and serratus anterior. Start with your right leg up and flexed, your left leg crossed over it with your ankle on your knee. Then with your left hand on your abdomen and your right hand behind the head, move from the down position, flat on the deck, and lift your right elbow to meet your left knee. Do these slowly to maximize constant tension and peak contraction. Pause at the top, not at the bottom. And again, don't pull on your neck!

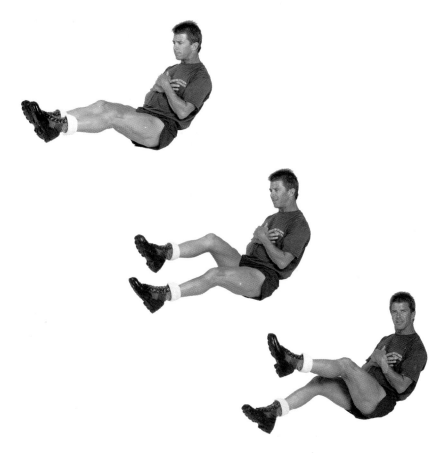

SITTING FLUTTER KICKS

With your butt on the deck, place your hands on your chest, legs up about six inches from the floor and start kicking. Keep your range of motion between six to 30 inches max. Again another fine way to prepare you for day-long ocean swims and underwater hydrographic reconnaissance missions.

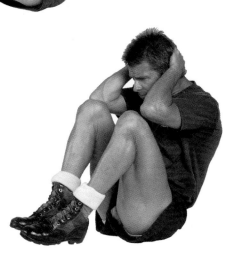

SITTING KNEE BENDERS

This is NOT an Atomic Situp! The major difference is that you start with your torso at a 45° angle to the ground. Extend your legs fully and keep your heels about six inches off the deck. Bring your knees in to meet your elbows. Extend your legs again. Repeat several times.

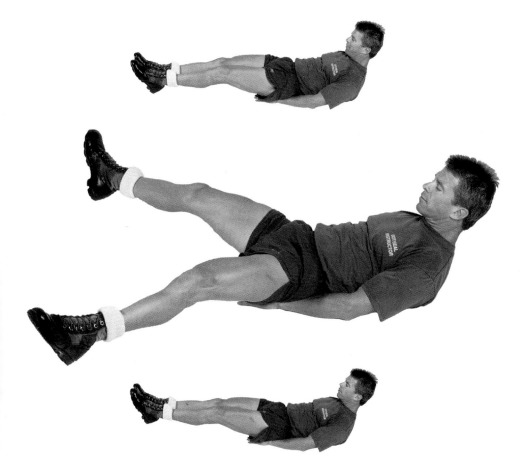

SCISSORS

Otherwise known as "Good Morning Darlings" at BUD/S, Scissors are another great way to strengthen your midsection. Lie on your back, cradling your torso with your arms as you did with the Leg Lever. Extend your legs out fully and keep your heels six inches off the deck. Open and close your legs as shown in the photo above. This exercise is counted in fours: open–close–open–close. One, two, three, ONE. One, two, three, TWO. One, two, three, THREE. Etc.

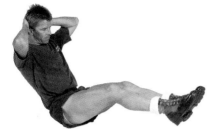

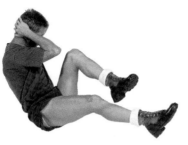

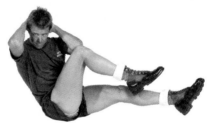

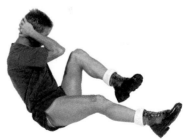

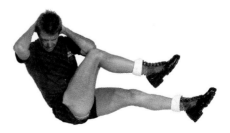

SITTING BICYCLES

The starting position is similar to the Sitting Knee Benders: hands behind head, torso at a 45° angle to the ground, legs fully extended, heels about six inches off the deck. Now, lift your knee as you twist your body and touch your knee with your opposite elbow. Think of your leg movement as if you were riding a bike. Alternate side-to-side in a continuous rhythmic motion.

77

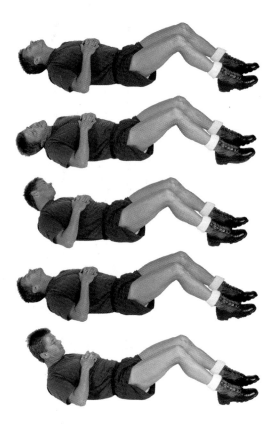

NECK ROTATIONS

It's not an ab exercise, but since you're on the deck now's as good time as any to do them. Strong neck muscles are important for one critical reason: to protect your neck and spine from sudden whip-type injuries. Think of the kind of things SEALs do and you will understand why: HALO parachuting from a C-130 transport, dropping 100 feet to the ocean from a Blackhawk helicopter, performing high-speed water insertions and retrievals. Any one of these can be potentially injurious if you have a weak neck. So don't forget to do these as part of your regular PT!

Keep it simple. Start on the deck. Legs comfortable as shown. Left-right-up-down. Reverse direction halfway through. Make that neck SEAL worthy! Hooyah!

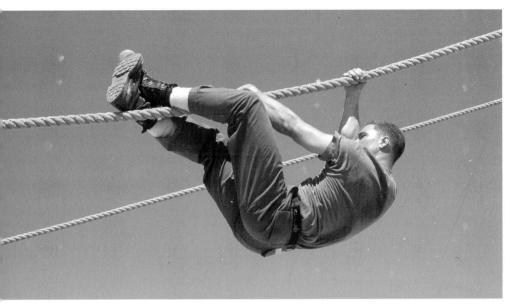

OBSTACLE
COURSE

The Obstacle Course is a major feature of SEAL training. It is another important component of the physical fitness readiness of each of the BUD/S students, and it builds confidence and competence physically.

A SEAL is made, not born. Watching SEALs fail, then gradually overcome the Obstacle Course is proof of this. There is a cross-section of people who enter SEAL training. There are great athletes. There are non-athletes, whose odds are against them but who make it nonetheless. In other words, a SEAL candidate is not necessarily a physical specimen. He could be someone with an average build, perhaps not uniquely successful as an athlete in high school, but somebody who has really got the grit and determination to stick with it.

The Obstacle Course is a measure of that spirit and determination that is an essential part of being a Navy SEAL. Are you ready? Then let's do it!

Parallel Bars → Low Wall → High Wall

NAVY
SEAL
O'
COURSE

Vaulting
Logs

↑

Spider
Wall

↑

Incline
Wall

↑

Tire
Sequence

↑

Rope
Swing

↑

Slide
for
Life
Tower

↑

↓

Barbed
Wire

↓

Cargo
Net

↓

Balance
Logs

↓

Hooyah
Logs

↓

Rope
Transfer

↓

The Dirty
Name

↓

More
Hooyah
Logs

← Burma Bridge ← The Weaver ←

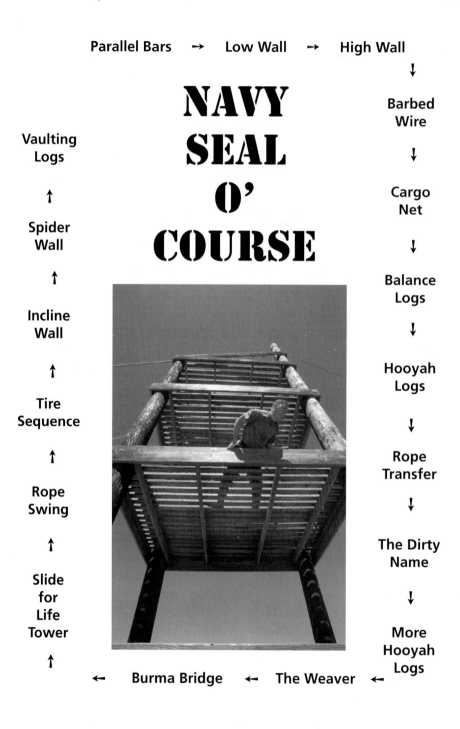

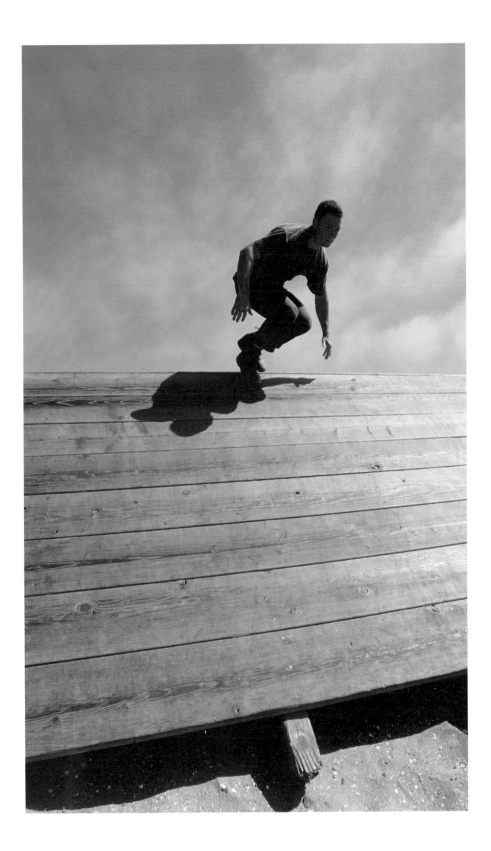

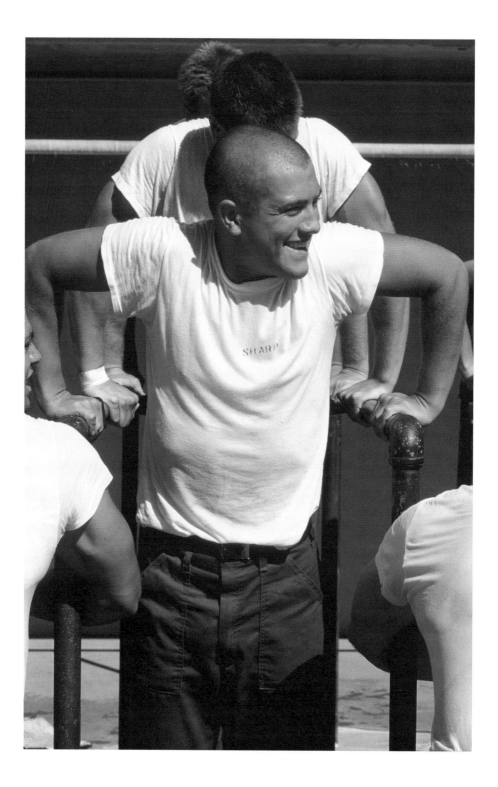

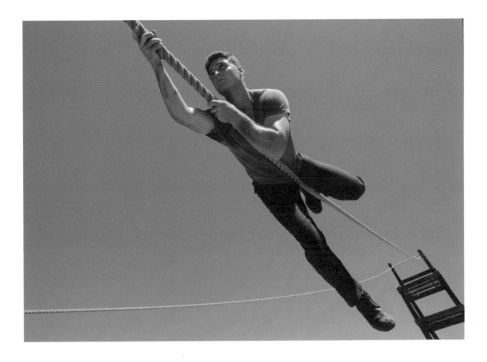

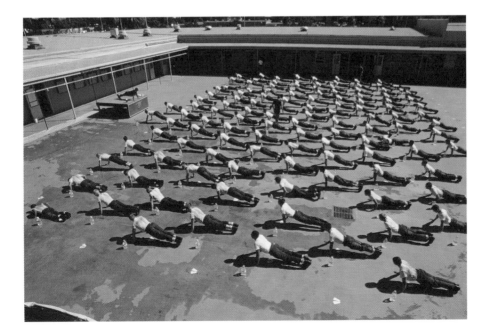

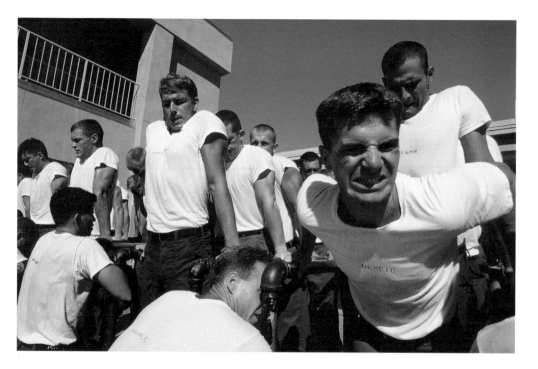

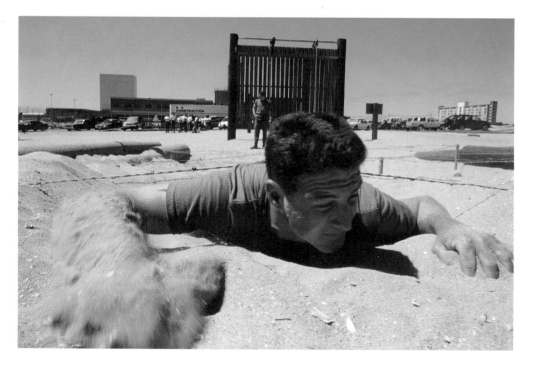

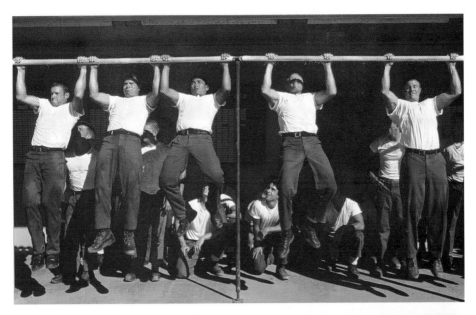

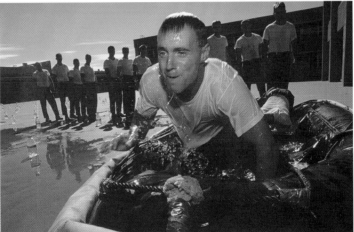

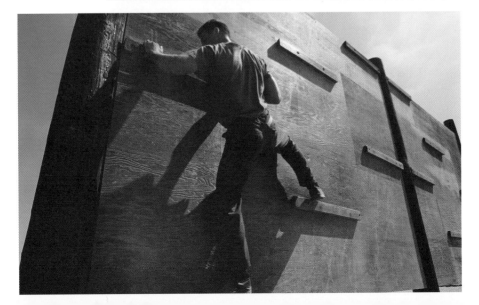

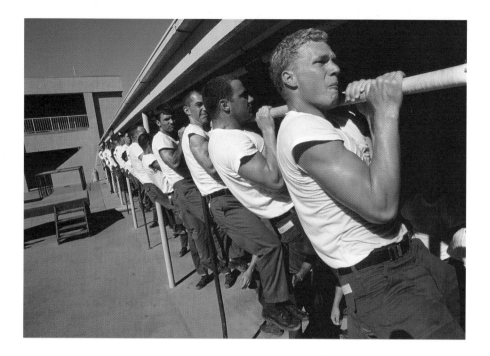

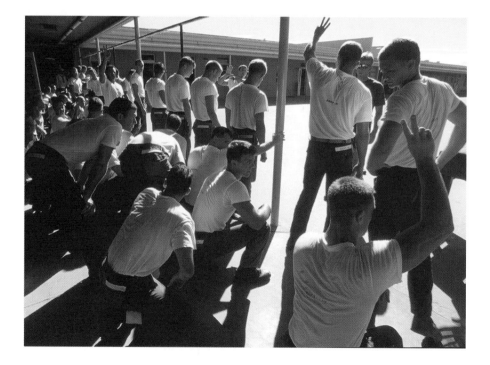

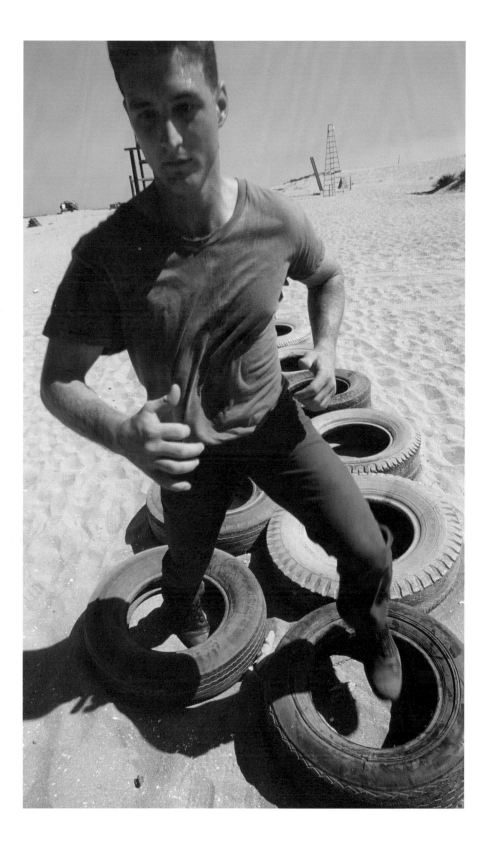

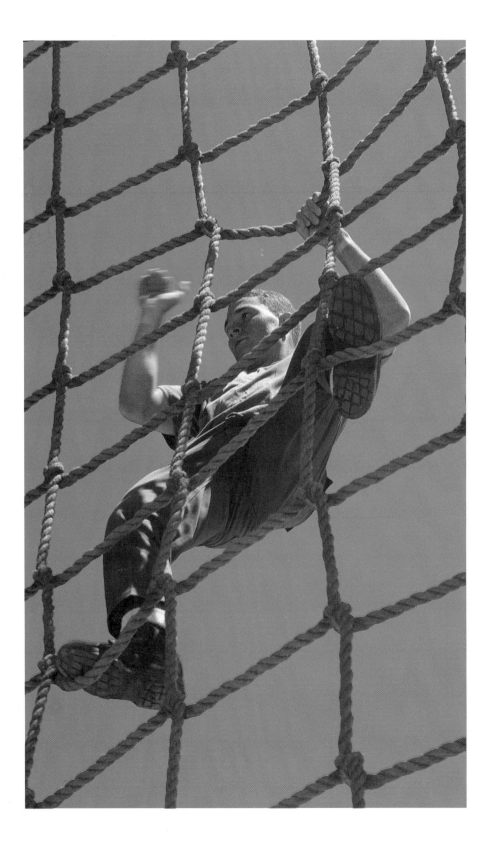

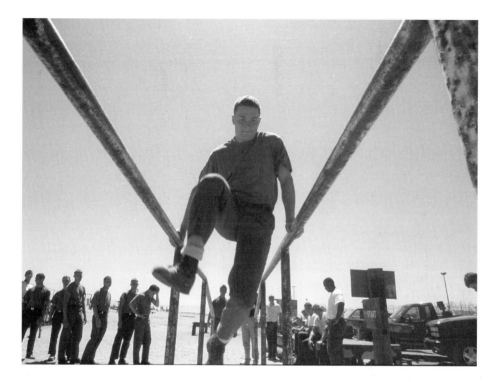

PARALLEL BARS

Traversing the Parallel Bars is like a moving Dip where you walk on your hands and bicycle pedal with your legs, or you can hop through on your hands. The length you must travel is about 20 feet. The bars are about five feet off the ground and they have an uphill section and then a flat section. You just work your way along. Easy day...so far. Then you run to the Low Wall.

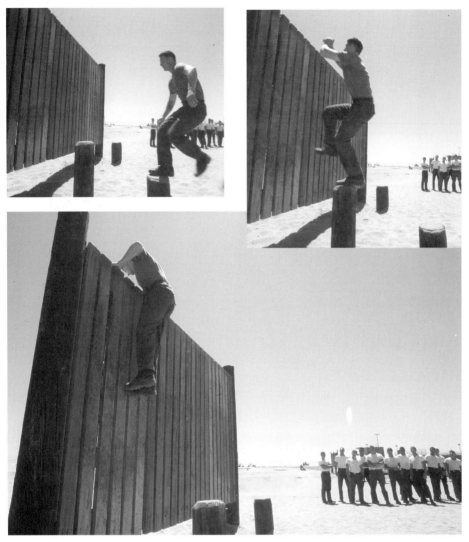

LOW WALL

The approach to the Low Wall is a series of telephone poles sawed down and stuck in the sand so they look like tree stumps. You leap from stump to stump and then launch yourself onto the Low Wall. It's only about 12 feet high. You jump onto it, grabbing the top with your hands, walking your feet up as you "mantle" or press up with your arms. Staying as low as you can and keeping your center of gravity down, you drop down on the other side.

Then there's a short run to the High Wall.

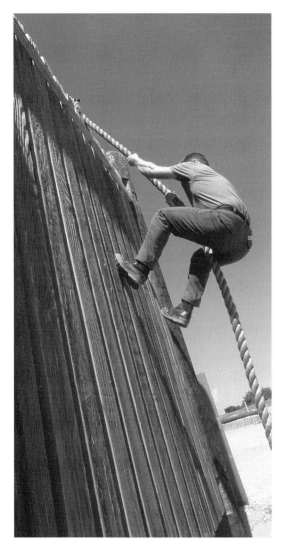

HIGH WALL

The face of the High Wall is sheathed with vertical boards. Suspended from the top of the Wall is an inviting and quite useful rope made of two-inch twisted manila hemp. Grabbing the rope, you climb up and hook a leg over the rail at the top, again keeping your center of gravity low, and swing over up onto the other side.

The key is to walk up the Wall, so you need to stay perpendicular to it. A lot of people tend to try to get upright—perpendicular to the ground—and that slows them down and their feet slide out from under them. But if you push away from it and just stay perpendicular to the Wall, you will succeed.

83

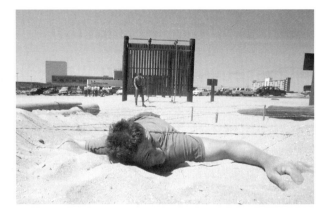

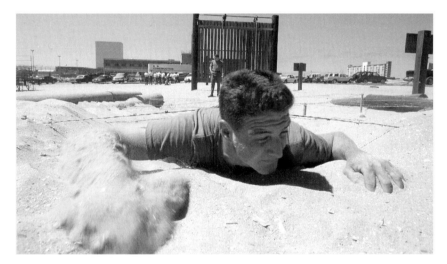

BARBED WIRE

Next you must crawl quickly underneath Barbed Wire. Barbed Wire is a feature of every traditional military obstacle course. The technique is to crawl on your belly, like a snake, and just pull yourself through, staying low and using your knees and elbows. You might take a little sand in your face here and there as you go through, but then again, this is SEAL training.

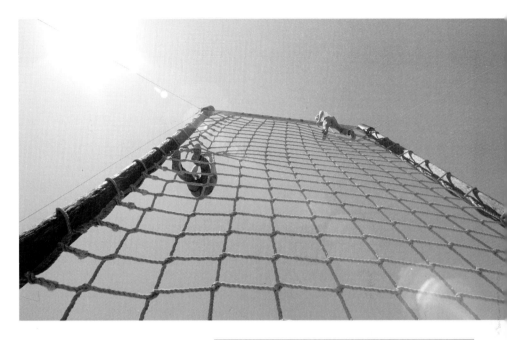

CARGO NET

Next you charge up the Cargo Net, over the rail, and down the other side. The Cargo Net rises to about 50 feet. The higher you go the more challenging it becomes. Although the Net is strung tightly and is replaced every six months, it still moves as you climb. The more SEALs on the Net, the more it moves and the more interesting it gets. SEALs learn to overcome their fear of heights quickly with the Cargo Net!

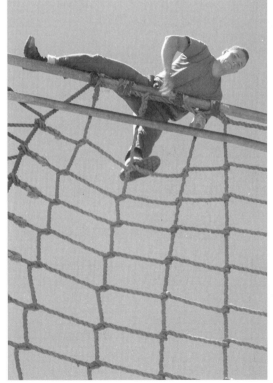

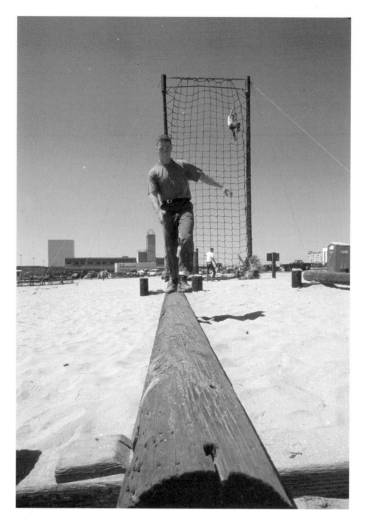

BALANCE LOGS

Next, there's a set of Balance Logs. There are three logs to negotiate. You go down one, turn left, and then go straight again. The logs are not fixed and they roll freely as you move along them, requiring you to keep your balance as you go.

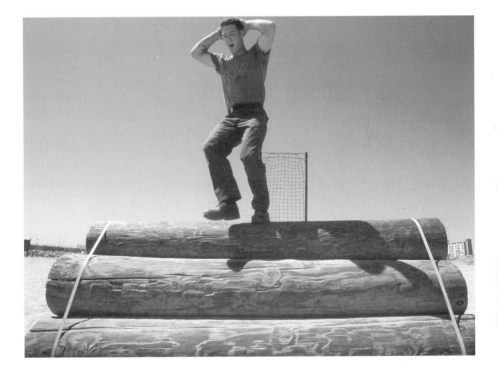

HOOYAH LOGS

The next obstacle is a set of ten logs stacked to form a pyramid. The SEALs call them Hooyah Logs because they run over them and say "Hooyah!" Although it's not required, many SEALs run them with their arms behind their heads...just for the challenge!

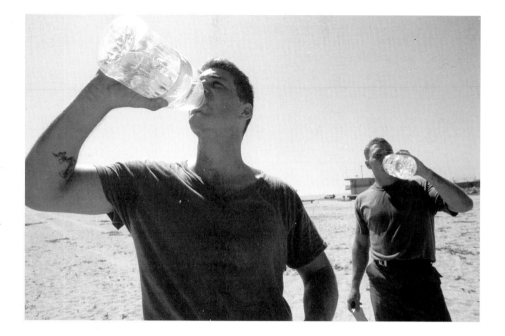

A WORD ON HYDRATION

Drinking plenty of water to stay hydrated is essential during work-outs. Stop and drink water between sets of pushups and pull-ups and at any other logical breaks during your workout as well as be-fore and after your workout—any time there is a break in the action.

Keep a supply of water handy. A used quart-sized sports drink bot-tle makes a great canteen.

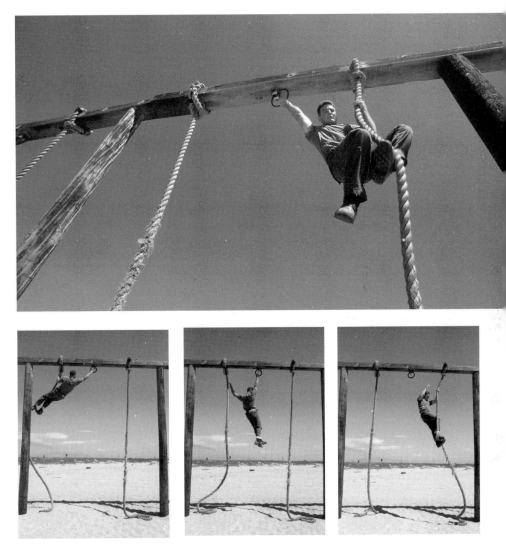

ROPE TRANSFER

Then there is the Rope Transfer. It's a real confidence and strength builder. The object is to climb up the rope to the left, grab the iron ring, then swing to the rope on the right and lower yourself down. On every obstacle proper technique is emphasized. When climbing and descending a rope, it is essential to maintain control to maximize speed and to minimize the risk of injury.

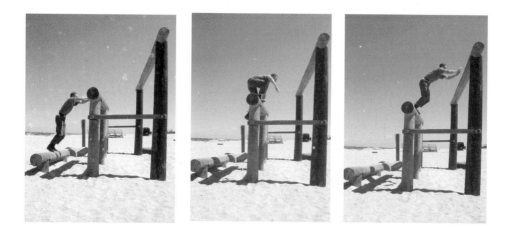

THE DIRTY NAME

When you see it, you know why it got its name! You vault off the bottom log, catching the middle log about hip level with your hands, and stand. If you think that's hard, you then have to launch yourself onto the higher log, catching it in the same manner with your hands at about hip level. Grabbing the high log you swing up and roll yourself over the top. Drop to the ground and you are done with the Dirty Name. At least for today.

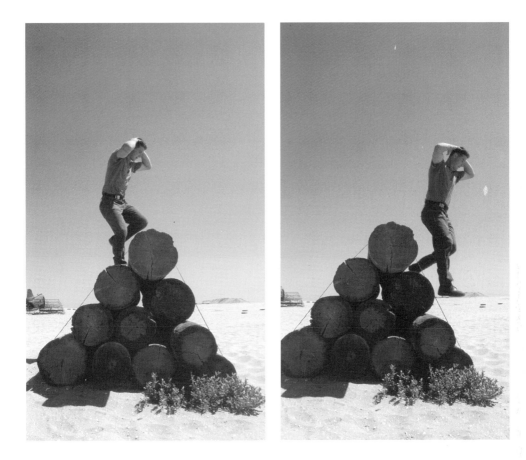

MORE HOOYAH LOGS

Then there are more Hooyah Logs to run over. Everyone likes the Hooyah Logs. It gives you a few moments to rest and recover some upper body strength before the next obstacle: the Weaver.

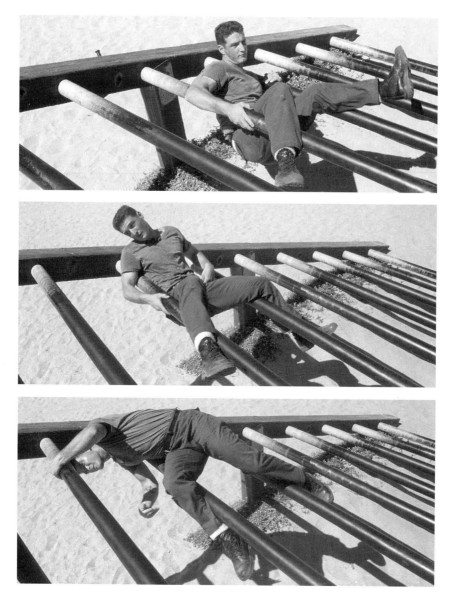

THE WEAVER

The Weaver is a really strange looking obstacle. It is a pyramid-shaped structure rising to about six feet. Built mostly of parallel iron pipes, it requires you to travel under one pipe and over the next, up to the high point and down the other side, weaving your way through it. Negotiating the Weaver takes a lot of coordination. SEALs find it's highly effective in slowing down overall completion times on the obstacle course...not that you needed help with that!

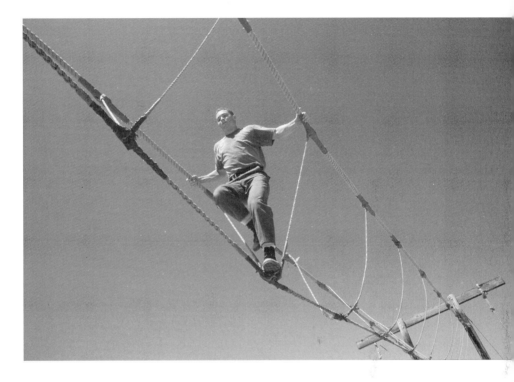

BURMA BRIDGE

Another classic military obstacle. The bridge extends about 75 feet in length and is accessed by a rope climb of about 12 feet. Traversing the Burma Bridge requires balance and coordination. The rope tends to pitch and sway as you go, the hand rails providing only a minimum of assistance. Descent from the Burma Bridge is also by rope.

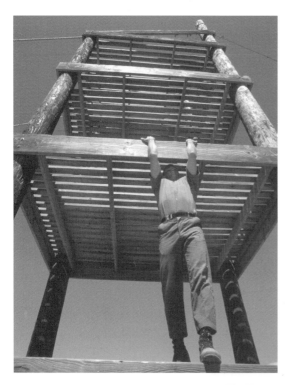

SLIDE FOR LIFE TOWER

The Slide for Life Tower is perhaps the most awesome and intimidating obstacle on the course. Here's a four-story tower (about 40 feet) that you first must ascend without the aid of ladders or steps, then you must descend from the top on one of two 100-foot ropes leading to the ground at a gentle angle.

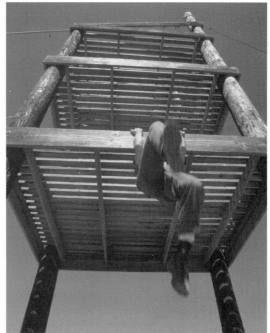

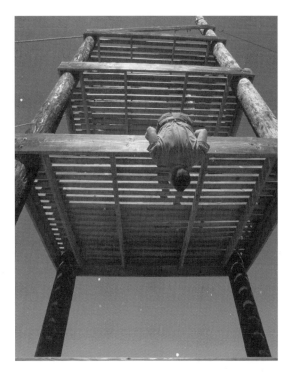

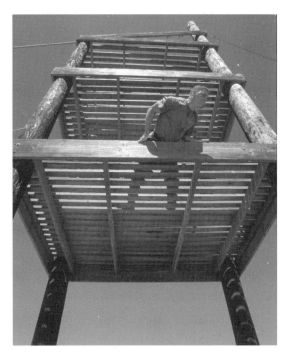

To climb up the tower, most SEALs use one of two techniques: the leg-over or the back flip. The leg-over is performed by first pulling yourself up by your arms (much like a pull-up) then throwing a leg over the top. You can use your heel to hook over the edge and then pull your body onto the next platform. It's certainly not a graceful technique but it gets the job done.

The back-flip method is just that. Facing outward, you grab the platform above you curl-up style and then using your momentum you flip yourself back over onto the next level. It is definitely the most efficient way to climb the Tower once perfected, but until then...practice at lower levels!

95

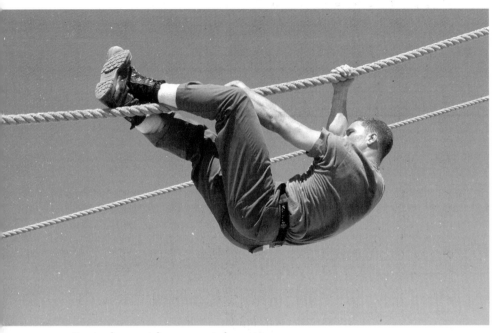

Rope descent banana style

Descent from the Tower on the Slide for Life is performed in one of two ways. You can descend "Banana Style," used during First and Second Phase of BUD/S, or you can descend "Commando Style" once you have entered Third Phase. Lowering yourself Banana Style is tough on the arms and legs. You are upside down and pulling yourself along hand over hand, with gravity working against you all the way down. Once you have mastered the Commando Style descent, it's much easier. Commando Style demands more agility and balance, but it is by far less exhausting. By Third Phase, SEAL candidates have had a lot of opportunity to hone their balance skills.

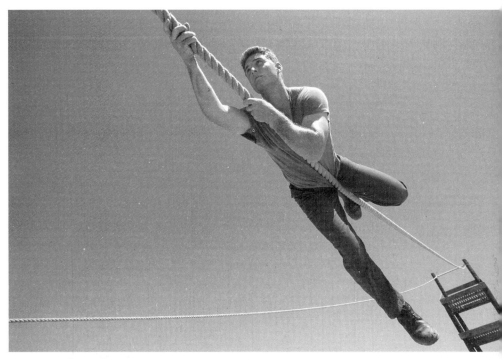

Commando style

SAFETY IS A #1 CONCERN

The Slide for Life Tower presents an excellent opportunity to mention safety. Many people ask, "Do people ever fall off the Tower?" Safety is a primary concern of the Navy SEALs, and especially of the instructors at BUD/S. A SEAL's job is dangerous enough, so why take unneeded risks? At the BUD/S Obstacle Course there is always a corpsman present as well as a safety officer. There is emergency transportation available, too. If for some reason a safety officer is not present, the Cargo Net and the Slide for Life Tower are omitted from the course that day.

If on the Slide for Life Tower a SEAL candidate thinks he is going to fall, he has been instructed to drop his legs, hang on with his hands, then fall feet first. It's soft sand and this controlled falling technique usually prevents injury. Still, some students fall without control, and the corpsman is prepared to provide aid if they do injure themselves.

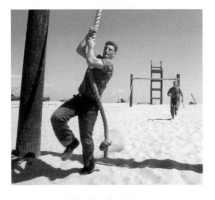

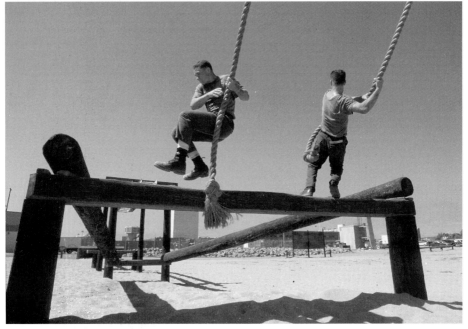

ROPE SWING

Once you have lowered yourself from the Slide for Life Tower, you proceed to the Rope Swing. The Rope Swing is harder than it looks. Using a rope, you swing from the sand to a log about four feet off the ground. You must land firmly on this log and let go of the rope quickly, or else you will find yourself eating sand. It's another example of proper technique winning over brute strength.

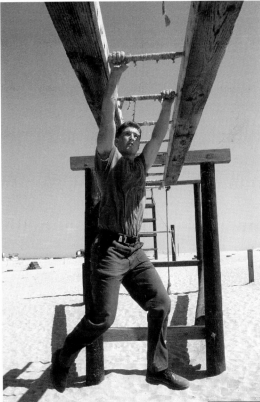

It's a quick walk down fixed logs to the Monkey Bars, which you travel hand over hand—just like when you were a kid. Only now you are in the hot sun and some other guy is coming up right behind you fast and it feels as if you've been doing this kind thing all day—because you have. Finishing the Monkey Bars you run along another fixed log (it's getting easier) and it's a quick sprint through the Tires.

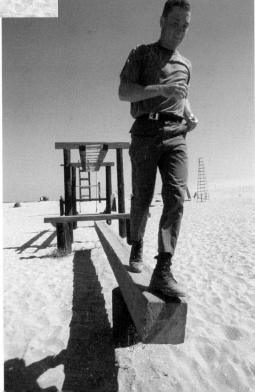

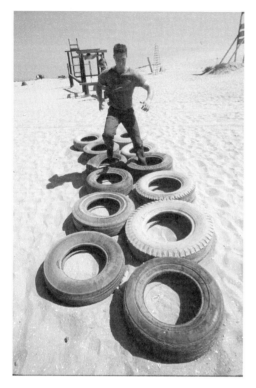

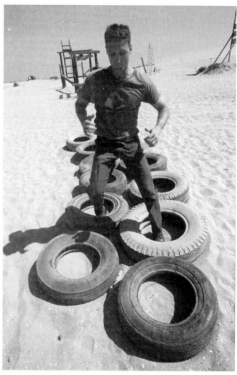

TIRE SEQUENCE

Hit the holes and not the rims as you make a dash for the Incline Wall.

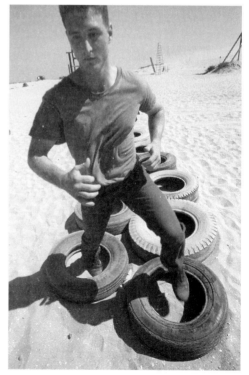

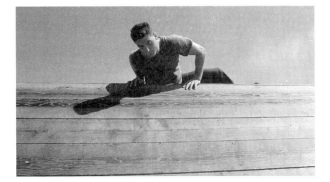

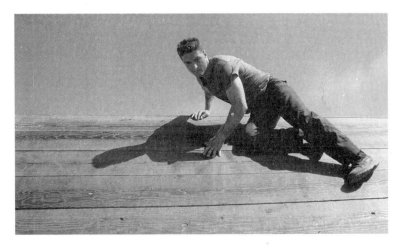

INCLINE WALL

Hop up and slide (or run down) the face. Piece of cake. Easy day. Wouldn't it be nice if all obstacles would be so gentle? Not so: Soon we will be burning our forearms on the Spider Wall.

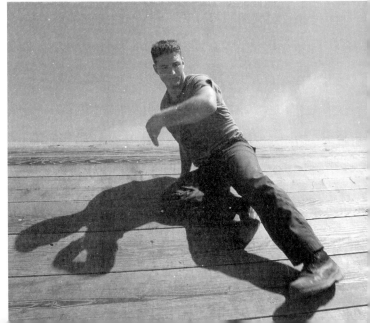

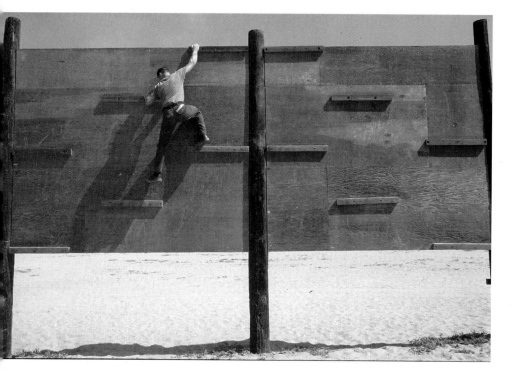

SPIDER WALL

The Spider Wall is quite similar to a climbing wall, and teaches similar skills. Balance, technique, agility—all come into play on the Spider Wall. The key is to use your legs to push yourself up rather than your arms. If you were to rely mostly on your arms on the Spider Wall your forearms would burn out before you completed the required traverse of the obstacle. Trust your legs and use your arms and hands as little as possible except for balance. You will feel great when you discover how easy it can be using proper climbing technique. We're almost done!

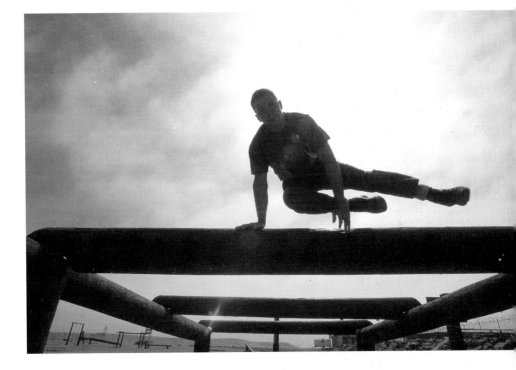

VAULTING LOGS

The last obstacle is the Vaulting Logs. They are a series of evenly spaced telephone poles parallel to the ground and about four feet high. The only rule: no touching with your legs or feet. You must hurdle over the logs quickly because time is running out.

Charge to the end. Give the BUD/S instructor and your classmates 20 perfect pushups. Stand up and say:

"Hooyah O'Course"

You're done! Easy day.

NUTRITION

Y ou can't achieve peak physical fitness without paying attention to what you eat. Strong dietary habits are critical both before entering BUD/S training and during the training program itself. Optimum performance is achieved by proper nutrient intake and is essential to receiving maximum performance output during exercise. Nutrition also promotes vital muscle and tissue growth and repair. The ideal diet provides all the nutrients that the body needs and supplies energy for exercise.

The Navy has developed a nutrition and weight control program to enable participants to vastly improve their health and fitness. The program deals with excess body fat and highlights the foods that will be most effective in helping you achieve your personal fitness goals. Used in conjunction with this or any physical conditioning regimen, this nutrition program will help you maintain and improve your health.

The following information on nutrition is essential for adopting healthy eating and exercise habits. Although the program is designed primarily as a weight management education tool, the Navy recommends it to all SEALs for the maintenance of long-term optimum health. The nutrition and diet program is successful only when used in conjunction with a physical conditioning program and is not to be used as a one-time, "quick fix" diet.

For example, a weight-loss program that reduces fat and incorporates complex carbohydrates but does not include exercise will ultimately fail. Similarly, increased exercise without a carefully monitored calorie intake will bring disappointing results. You need to consume a great amount of complex carbohydrates to provide the energy you need to sustain a strenuous physical program at BUD/S.

A healthy body fat percentage for men is 14 to 16 percent; for women, 24 to 26 percent.

Before starting a nutrition or a weight-control program, it is essential to understand the way our bodies process the foods we eat.

WHAT IS NUTRITION?

Nutrition is the science of nourishment, the study of nutrients and the process by which organisms use them. In other words, nutrition is the way our bodies get energy from the food we eat. So the old saying, "You are what you eat" may not be far from the truth, considering the performance of the body is directly related to how we fuel ourselves. The study of nutrition has proven that poor nutritional habits have a profound effect on physical and mental capabilities and affect all functions of the body. Without the most fundamental of nutrients, including water, the body quickly begins to deteriorate.

Good nutrition is fundamental to every living organism on the earth in order to grow and function properly. There are six nutrients derived from food: carbohydrates, protein, and fat, which provide the body with calories; and vitamins, minerals, and water, which provide no calories. It is important to

After exhaustive exercise, it takes at least 20 hours to completely restore muscle energy.

note that while carbohydrates and proteins supply the body with four calories each per gram, fat contributes nine calories per gram—more than double. Therefore, it is important to monitor fat intake when maintaining or losing weight. Similarly, a diet and exercise program must incorporate carbohydrates that provide the body with the energy needed to sustain an exercise regimen.

Carbohydrates are sugars and starches in food and are derived from the plant kingdom. Typically, carbohydrates are called either simple or complex and provide the body with most of its fuel. Examples of complex carbohydrates include bread, rice, pasta, potatoes, cereals, and whole grains. Simple carbohydrates include fruits and vegetables. Refined simple sugars are found in candy, cakes, cookies, sodas, etc. and provide a quick source of energy. Some carbohydrates, such as fruits and vegetables, are also rich in dietary fiber, another chief element of a healthy diet.

A high carbohydrate diet is essential to maintaining energy during heavy training.

Dietary fiber is found only in plant food and is the "indigestible" part of the plant. So although fiber is edible, it is not digested or absorbed by humans. Similarly, fiber itself is calorie-free although typically foods rich in fiber usually contain calories. Fiber is made up of two types: soluble and insoluble. Soluble fiber lowers cholesterol levels. Its sources include fruits and vegetables, especially apples, oranges, carrots, oat bran, barley, and beans. Insoluble fiber increases the bulk of food thereby speeding the passage of food through the digestive tract. Insoluble fiber is found in fruits with edible skins, whole grains and breads, and whole grain cereals. Although 25 to 30 grams of fiber per day is recommended, statistics show that most Americans fail to consume this recommended daily allowance and take in only 10 to 15 grams per day.

Protein is essential to the human body. Protein functions to repair and build tissues, provide a structural role in all body tissues and contributes to the formation of enzymes, hormones, and antibodies. Protein consists of amino acids that are sometimes called the "building blocks" of protein. Protein in the diet is broken down into amino acids during digestion. Complete proteins are foods containing large amounts of essential amino acids. Complete proteins are found in animal proteins including beef, chicken, pork, fish, eggs, milk, and cheese. There are also incomplete proteins, which, as their name implies, are deficient in one or more of the eight essential amino acids. Incomplete proteins are derived from non-animal sources such as legumes including soybeans, peanuts, peas, beans and lentils, grains, and vegetables.

Fat. Perhaps the most talked about issue recently has been the presence of fat in our diets. Fat comes from the oils found in food and is stored in the body as triglycerides, which are more commonly known as body fat. Fat is found in vegetable oils, butter, shortening, lard, margarine, and animal foods such as beef, chicken, and diary products. The popular misconception is that all fat is bad. Adults require a minimum of 15 to 25 grams of fat daily. Fat manufactures antibodies to fight disease, serves as carriers of certain vitamins, protects vital organs, and insulates the body against environmental temperature changes. In addition, fat lines and insulates neurons or nerves, which allow all neural information to move through the brain and the body. We would not be able to move or think without the presence of fat. There are three different kinds of fat: polyunsaturated, monosaturated, and saturated.

FINDING THE RIGHT BALANCE

How does all of this translate to our personal fitness and weight loss? Remember that while carbohydrates and proteins produce only 4 calories per gram, fat provides the body with 9 calories per gram. There are 3,500 calories on one pound of fat tissue. When someone consumes 3,500 calories more than they burn, they gain one pound of fat. Similarly, when they use 3,500 calories more than they consume, they lose one pound of fat. A healthy body fat percentage for men is 14 to 16 percent; for women, 24 to 26 percent.

Although all three—carbohydrates, protein, and fat—are sources of energy nutrients, carbohydrates are the preferred source of energy for physical activity. After exhaustive exercise, it takes at least 20 hours to completely restore muscle energy, assuming that 600 grams of carbohydrates are consumed per day. A high carbohydrate diet is essential to maintaining energy during successive days of heavy training when energy stores before each training session become progressively lower.

The popular misconception is that all fat is bad.

The best sources of complex carbohydrates are bread, crackers, cereal, beans, pasta, potatoes, rice, fruits, and vegetables. *You should consume at least four servings of these food groups per day when training.*

Stay hydrated. In addition, frequent water intake is crucial. It is important to stay hydrated and consume water prior to feeling thirsty. Drink at least four quarts of water daily, staying away from alcohol, caffeine, and tobacco, which increase your body's need for water.

Although conditioned to eat three meals a day, ideally we should get calories from smaller meals spread evenly throughout the day.

Good nutritional habits should not be limited to a specified training period but must become a lifetime commitment. Although we have been conditioned to think that eating three square meals per day is healthy, ideally calories should be spread evenly throughout the day with smaller meals that may occur three, four, five, or six times a day. The amount of meals and the numbers of hours in between eating should be based on each particular lifestyle.

Skipping meals, especially breakfast, is strongly inadvisable. According to research, approximately 90 percent of people with a weight problem skip at least one or two meals daily with breakfast being the most frequently missed. Skipping meals causes the metabolism to lower itself to conserve energy. It also promotes overeating in the evening after a meal has been skipped during the day. However, research shows that metabolism increases by 50 percent after eating breakfast.

Metabolism increases by 50 percent after eating breakfast.

It is strongly recommended that you keep a log of everything you have consumed, including fluids, during the day. Record each meal or snack along with the time of day. In this way, your progress will be accurately marked and serve as a vital tool in advancing your physical state of well-being.

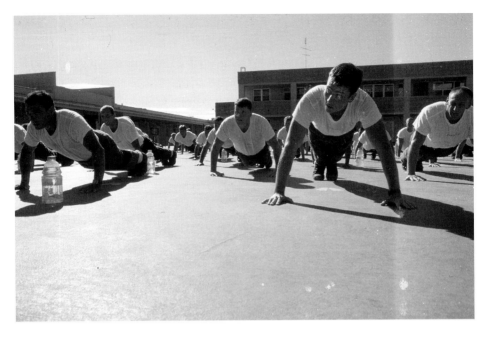

PREPARE YOURSELF
FOR THE NAVY SEALS

The following section has been excerpted from the BUD/S Warning Order, an official publication of Naval Special Warfare designed to provide information for both civilians and naval personnel interested in applying to BUD/S training. This excerpt focuses on physical fitness readiness. To get a complete copy of the BUD/S Warning Order, contact your Navy recruiter (FYI: A warning order is a Navy term for an informational brief which describes a mission and how it is to be completed.)

The following workouts are designed for two categories of people: Category I are those future BUD/S students who have never or have not recently been on a routine PT program, and Category II is designed for high school and college athletes that have had a routine PT program. Usually, athletes who require a high level of cardiovascular activity are in Category II. Swimming, running, and wrestling are good examples of such sports.

WORKOUT FOR CATEGORY I

The majority of the physical activities you will be required to perform during your six months of training at BUD/S will involve running. The intense amount of running can lead to stress injuries of the lower extremities in trainees who arrive not physically prepared to handle the activities. Swimming, bicycling, and lifting weights will prepare you for some of the activities at BUD/S, but ONLY running can prepare your lower extremities for the majority of the activities. You should also run in boots to prepare your legs for the everyday running in boots at BUD/S. (Boots should be of a lightweight variety, i.e., Bates Lights, Hi-Tec, etc.)

The goal of the Category I student is to work up to 16 miles per week of running. After you have achieved that goal, then and only then should you continue on to the Category II goal of 30 miles per week. Remember, Category I is a nine-week buildup program. Follow the workout as best you can and you will be amazed at the progress you will make.

RUNNING SCHEDULE I

WEEK #1 and 2:	2 miles/day, 8:30 pace, M/W/F	(6 miles/week)
WEEK #3:	No running. High risk of stress fractures.	
WEEK #4:	3 miles/day, M/W/F	(9 miles/wk)
WEEKS #5 and 6:	2/3/4/2 miles, M/Tu/Th/F	(11 miles/wk)
WEEKS #7 and 8:	4/4/5/3 miles, M/Tu/Th/F	(16 miles/wk)
WEEK #9:	same as weeks #7, 8	(16 miles/wk)

PHYSICAL TRAINING SCHEDULE I
(Mon/Wed/Fri)

SETS OF REPETITIONS		SETS OF REPETITIONS	
WEEK #1:	4X15 PUSHUPS 4X20 SITUPS 3X3 PULL-UPS	WEEKS #5, 6:	6X25 PUSHUPS 6X25 SITUPS 2X8 PULL-UPS
WEEK #2:	5X20 PUSHUPS 5X20 SITUPS 3X3 PULL-UPS	WEEKS #7,8:	6X30 PUSHUPS 6X30 SITUPS 2X10 PULL-UPS
WEEKS #3, 4:	5X25 PUSHUPS 5X25 SITUPS 3X4 PULL-UPS	WEEK #9:	6X30 PUSHUPS 6X30 SITUPS 3X10 PULL-UPS

Note: For best results, alternate exercises. Do a set of pushups, then a set of situps, followed by a set of pull-ups, immediately, with no rest.

SWIMMING SCHEDULE I
(sidestroke with no fins, 4 to 5 days a week)

WEEKS #1, 2:	Swim continuously for 15 min.
WEEKS #3, 4:	Swim continuously for 20 min.
WEEKS #5, 6:	Swim continuously for 25 min.
WEEKS #7, 8:	Swim continuously for 30 min.
WEEK #9:	Swim continuously for 35 min.

Note: If you do not have access to a pool, ride a bicycle for twice as long as you would swim. If you do have access to a pool, swim every day that it's available. Four to five days a week and 200 meters in one

113

session is your initial workup goal. Also, you want to develop your sidestroke on both the left and the right side. Try to swim 50 meters in one minute or less.

WORKOUT FOR CATEGORY II

Category II is a more intense workout designed for those who have been involved with a routine PT schedule or those who have completed the requirements of Category I. DO NOT ATTEMPT THIS WORKOUT SCHEDULE UNLESS YOU CAN COMPLETE THE WEEK #9 LEVEL OF CATEGORY I WORKOUTS.

RUNNING SCHEDULE II

	M/Tu/Th/F/Sat.	TOTAL
WEEKS #1, 2:	(3/5/4/5/2) miles	19 miles/week
WEEKS #3, 4:	(4/5/6/4/3) miles	22 miles/week
WEEK #5:	(5/5/6/4/4) miles	24 miles/week
WEEK #6:	(5/6/6/6/4) miles	27 miles/week

Note: Beyond week #6, it is not necessary to increase the distance of the runs; work on the speed of your six-mile runs and try to get them down to 7:30 per mile or lower. If you wish to increase the distance of your runs, do it gradually: no more than one mile per day increase for every week beyond week #6.

PHYSICAL TRAINING SCHEDULE II
(Mon/Wed/Fri)

	SETS OF REPETITIONS			SETS OF REPETITIONS	
WEEKS #1, 2:	6X30	PUSHUPS	WEEKS #3, 4:	10X20	PUSHUPS
	6X35	SITUPS		10X25	SITUPS
	3X10	PULL-UPS		4X10	PULL-UPS
	3X20	DIPS		10X15	DIPS
WEEK #5:	15X20	PUSHUPS	WEEK #6:	20X20	PUSHUPS
	15X25	SITUPS		20X25	SITUPS
	4X12	PULL-UPS		5X12	PULL-UPS
	15X15	DIPS		20X15	DIPS

These workouts are designed for long-distance muscle endurance. Muscle fatigue will gradually take a longer and longer time to develop doing high-repetition workouts. For best results, alternate exercises each set, in order to rest that muscle group for a short time. The below listed workouts are provided for varying your workouts once you have met the Category I and II standards.

PYRAMID WORKOUTS

You can do this with any exercise. The object is to slowly build up to a goal, then build back down to the beginning of the workout. For instance, pull-ups, situps, pushups, and dips can be alternated as in the above workouts, but this time choose a number to be your goal and

115

build up to that number. Each number counts as a set. Work your way up and down the pyramid.

For example, say your goal is "5."

Start at the base of the pyramid on the left side with one pull-up, working your way up to five and then ending on the right base of the pyramid with one again.

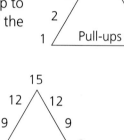

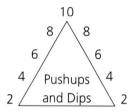

SWIMMING WORKOUTS II
(4-5 days/week)

WEEKS #1, 2:	Swim continuously for 35 min.
WEEKS #3, 4:	Swim continuously for 45 min. with fins.
WEEK #5:	Swim continuously for 60 min. with fins.
WEEK #6:	Swim continuously for 75 min. with fins.

Note: At first, to reduce initial stress on your foot muscles when starting with fins, alternate swimming 1,000 meters with fins and 1,000 meters without them. Your goal should be to swim 50 meters in 45 seconds or less.

STRETCH PHYSICAL TRAINING (PT)

Since Monday, Wednesday, and Friday are devoted to PT, it is wise to devote at least 20 minutes on Tuesday, Thursday, and Saturday to stretching. You should always stretch for at least 15 minutes before any workout; however, just stretching the previously worked muscles will make you more flexible and less likely to get injured. A good way to start stretching is to start at the top and go to the bottom. Stretch to tightness, not to pain; hold for 10 to 15 seconds. DO NOT BOUNCE. Stretch every muscle in your body from the neck to the calves, concentrating on your thighs, hamstrings, chest, back, and shoulders.

NUTRITION

Proper nutrition is extremely important now and especially when you arrive at BUD/S. You must make sure you receive the necessary nutrients to obtain maximum performance output during exercise and to promote muscle/tissue growth and repair. The proper diet provides all the nutrients for the body's needs and supplies energy for exercise. It also promotes growth and repair of tissue and regulates the body processes. The best source of complex carbohydrates are potatoes, pasta, rice, fruits, and vegetables. These types of foods are your best sources of energy.

The majority of carbohydrates should come from complex carbohydrate foods that include bread, crackers, cereal, beans, peas, starchy vegetables, and other whole grain or enriched grain products. Fruits are also loaded with carbohydrates. During training, more than four servings of these food groups should be consumed daily.

Water intake is vital; stay hydrated. You should be consuming up to four quarts of water daily. Drink water before you get thirsty! Supplemental intake of vitamins, as well, has not been proven to be beneficial. If you are eating a well-balanced diet, there is no need to take vitamins.

TRAINING TABLE CONCEPT

NUTRIENT	INTAKE
Carbohydrates	50-70% of calories
Protein	10-15% of calories
Fats	20-30% of calories

In each Phase of BUD/S, students must meet a series of physical fitness standards before proceeding to the next Phase. As you look at the following charts, you will be impressed by the strenuous standards of the Navy SEALs.

PHYSICAL FITNESS STANDARDS

Physical Evolution	Required Time

FIRST PHASE

50 meter underwater swim	Pass/Fail
Underwater knot tying	Pass/Fail
Drown Proofing Test	Pass/Fail
Basic lifesaving test	Pass/Fail
1200 meter pool swim with fins	45 min.
1 mile bay swim with fins	50 min.
1 mile ocean swim with fins	50 min.
1 1/2 mile ocean swim with fins	70 min.
2 mile ocean swim with fins	95 min.
Obstacle course	15 min.
4-mile timed run	32 min.

FIRST PHASE: POST HELL WEEK

2000 meter pool swim without fins	Completion
1 1/2 mile night bay swim with fins	Completion
2 mile ocean swim with fins	85 min.
4-mile timed run	32 min.
Obstacle course	13 min.

Physical Evolution	Required Time

SECOND PHASE

2 mile ocean swim with fins	80 min.
4-mile timed run in boots	31 min.
Obstacle course	10 min. 30 sec.
3 1/2 mile ocean swim with fins	Completion
5 1/2 mile ocean swim with fins	Completion

THIRD PHASE

Obstacle Course	10 min.
4-mile timed run in boots	30 min.
14 mile run	Completion
2 mile ocean swim with fins	75 min.

Students must also meet academic standards before graduating from BUD/S. For officers, scores must be 80% or above; for enlisted men, 70% or above.

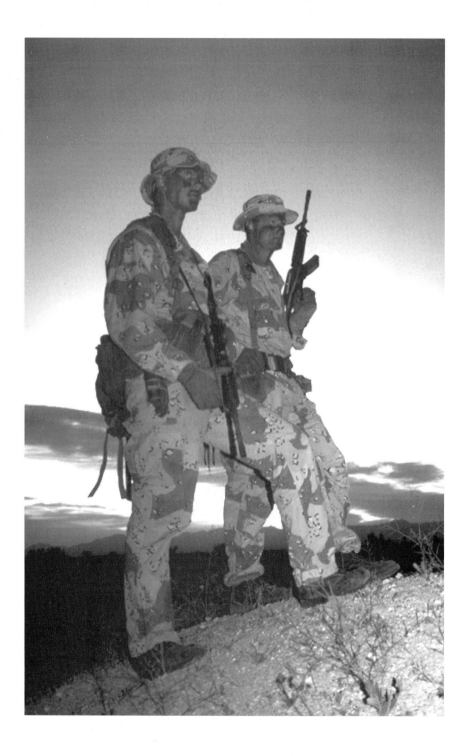

The Five Star NAVY SEAL Total Body Workout

The following workout schedules have been developed by the editors at Five Star Fitness. They incorporate the exercises you'll find in this book, and have been tailored to meet a variety of fitness levels. It is our hope that these guidelines will bring you to a level of fitness appropriate for your age and health.

Keep in mind, it is *highly* recommended that you seek the advice of proper personnel who can design a training program suitable to your individual needs and that you consult a physician before commencing any new exercise program or before intensifying any existing exercise program. Also consider these important factors which may affect your fitness regimen:

- Your age
- Your recent physical fitness activities
- Any medical conditions
- Any related health concerns (smoking, heavy alcohol drinking, weight issues)

The bottom line: take your health seriously!

LEVEL 1: BASIC TRAINING

Approximate time for the workout: 1 hour.

Ideal starting point. Nice and easy. You'll get familiar with the exercises and within a few weeks, you'll feel a level of confidence to move to Level 2.

LEVEL 2: JUNIOR UDT

Approximate time for the workout: 1 hour.

Moving up, you are still getting used to a regular fitness routine. You're introduced to a variety of pull-up variations, and your ab workout is intensified. Running or swimming is required in the cardio portion of your workout.

LEVEL 3: FUTURE SEAL

Approximate time for the workout: 1.5 hours.

It's *almost* time to take the training wheels off. Time for a couple more pushup variations and you're introduced to rope climbing. If you have trouble finding a rope to climb, well...look harder! Rope climbing is a phenomenal way to build upper body strength. Warmups now include running, not walking. If pressed for time, substitute 15 minutes of continuous jumping jacks for the mile run.

LEVEL 4: FIT AS A FROGMAN

Approximate time for the workout: 2 hours.

Solid, heavy duty PT for the rest of us. If you achieve this fitness level alone you're going to be in fantastic shape. Frogmen love the water, so you might want to alternate your swimming and running as cardio workouts. Learn the proper swim strokes: check out *The Com-*

plete Guide to Navy SEAL Fitness by Stewart Smith for a thorough presentation of swimming in the Navy SEALs.

LEVEL 5: BRAVING BUD/S

Approximate time for the workout: 2 hours.

This is a combination of PT exercises you'll find the BUD/S candidates performing at the Naval Special Warfare Center. All stops are out as you punch through Grinder PT with the best of them. Too easy? Add sets, increase reps. Still too easy....check out recruiting info and apply for BUD/S...once there, your instructors will find a variety of ways to challenge you physically and mentally.

To determine your beginning level, use the following suggested guidelines:

LEVEL	1	2	3	4	5
Pushups (in 2 mins)	1-10	11-20	21-30	31-50	51+
Pull-ups (max)	0-3	4-9	10-15	16-25	26+
Situps (in 2 mins)	5-15	16-25	26-40	41-60	61+
Running (1 mile)	can't do it	12:00	10:00	9:00	8:00
Swimming (.25 mile)	can't do it	20:00	15:00	12:00	10:00

If any or all of your abilities fall within a category above, stick with that category. For example, if you can do 20 pushups, but can't run a mile, start at Level 1. If you can do 50 situps, but only 6 pull-ups, start at Level 2. OR mix Levels. For example, your upper body PT may be Level 2 and your Ab PT may be Level 3. Either way, be consistent with your choices. Don't change Levels up and down and up again, for instance.

Remember to stick with chosen workout Level for at least 4 weeks. If it gets too easy (you'll know when) increase the number of reps per exercise. If it's still too easy, add another set. Whatever you do, stick with the schedule!

Check out our website, www.getfitnow.com, for a discussion area relating to this workout. Here you'll find an opportunity to ask questions and get feedback, as well as review questions and discussions of others following the *Five Star Navy SEAL Total Body Workout.*

WEEKLY WORKOUT SCHEDULE

Sunday	Monday	Tuesday	Wednesday	Thursday	Friday	Saturday
OFF	Warmup	Warmup	Warmup	Warmup	Warmup	Warmup
	Stretch	Stretch	Stretch	Stretch	Stretch	Stretch
	Upper Body PT	Lower Body PT	Upper Body PT	Lower Body PT	Upper Body PT	
	Pull-up PT		Pull-up PT		Pull-up PT	
	AB PT	AB PT	AB PT	AB PT	AB PT	
	Body Builders	Body Builders	Body Builders	Body Builders	Body Builders	
	Cardio	Cardio	Cardio	Cardio	Cardio	
	Rope Climb	Rope Climb	Rope Climb	Rope Climb	Rope Climb	

RUN

Level	Miles
1	1
2	2
3	3
4	4
5	5

Note: Stick with workout level for 4 weeks. If it gets too easy (you'll know when), increase the number of reps per exercise. If it's still too easy, add another set. Stick with the schedule!

LEVEL 1

Warmup

Walk/Jog	15 min

Stretch

Hurdler	Left and Right (L/R) 30 sec
or	
Modified Hurdler	L/R 30 sec
Sitting Head to Knee	30 sec
Back Rollers (optional)	30 sec
Butterfly	30 sec
Groin Stretch	30 sec
ITB Stretch	L/R 30 sec
Swimmer Stretch	30 sec
Triceps Stretch	L/R 15 sec
Press-Press-Fling	10
Up Back and Over	10
Trunk Rotations	4
Trunk Benders	5

Upper Body

Pushup Regular	10
Arm Haulers	10

Abdominals

Situp	10
Leg Lever	10
Atomic Situp	5
Back Flutter Kick	10
Crunches Heel in Close	10
Crunches Legs Up	10
Cross Leg Situp	L/R 6
Sitting Flutter Kick	5
Sitting Knee Benders	5
Scissors	10
Sitting Bicycles	10
Neck Rotations	L/R 15 Up and Down 20

These exercises are optional or substitutes

LEVEL 1

Lower Body

Lunges	10
Squat Leaps	5

Pull-ups

Pull-up Regular	max
Pull-up Reverse	max
Dips	max

Cardio

Treadmill: Walking (miles) or	1.5
Swimming (miles)	0.25

Other

Eight Count Body Builder	5

LEVEL 2

Warmup	
Walk/Jog	15 min

Stretch	
Hurdler	L/R 30 sec
or	
Modified Hurdler	L/R 30 sec
Sitting Head to Knee	30 sec
Back Rollers (optional)	30 sec
Butterfly	30 sec
Groin Stretch	30 sec
ITB Stretch	L/R 30 sec
Swimmer Stretch	30 sec
Triceps Stretch	L/R 15 sec
Press-Press-Fling	10
Up Back and Over	10
Trunk Rotations	4
Trunk Benders	5

Upper Body	
Pushup Regular	10 x 2
Arm Haulers	15

Abdominals	
Situp	25
Leg Lever	25
Atomic Situp	10
Back Flutter Kick	20
Crunches Heel in Close	10 x 2
Crunch Legs Up	10 x 2
Cross Leg Situp	L/R 12
Sitting Flutter Kick	10
Sitting Knee Benders	10
Scissors	20
Sitting Bicycles	20
Neck Rotations	L/R 15 U/D 20

These exercises are optional or substitutes

LEVEL 2

Lower Body

Lunges	15
Squat Leaps	10
Side Lunge	5

Pull-ups

Pull-up Regular	max x 2
Pull-up Wide	max
Pull-up Reverse	max x 2
Pull-up Close	max
Cliffhangers	max
Dips	max x 2

Cardio

Treadmill: Running (miles)	1
or	
Swimming (miles)	0.5

Other

Eight Count Body Builder	10

LEVEL 3

Warmup	
Running	1 mile

Stretch	
Hurdler	L/R 30 sec
or	
Modified Hurdler	L/R 30 sec
Sitting Head to Knee	30 sec
Back Rollers (optional)	30 sec
Butterfly	30 sec
Groin Stretch	30 sec
ITB Stretch	L/R 30 sec
Swimmer Stretch	30 sec
Triceps Stretch	L/R 15 sec
Press-Press-Fling	10
Up Back and Over	10
Trunk Rotations	4
Trunk Benders	5

Upper Body	
Pushup Regular	15 x 2
Pushup Triceps	7 x 2	⟩ (x4)
Pushup Dive Bomber	10 x 2
Arm Haulers	20

Abdominals	
Situp	25 x 2
Leg Lever	25 x 2
Atomic Situp	10 x 2
Back Flutter Kick	20 x 2
Crunches Heel in Close	20 x 2
Crunches Extended Leg	20 x 2
Cross Leg Situp	L/R 12 x 2
Sitting Flutter Kick	10 x 2
Sitting Knee Benders	10 x 2
Scissors	20 x 2
Sitting Bicycles	20 x 2
Neck Rotations	L/R 15 U/D 20

These exercises are optional or substitutes

LEVEL 3

Lower Body

Lunges	20
Squat Leaps	15
Side Lunge	10
Star Jumpers	5

Pull-ups

Pull-up Regular	4 x 2
Pull-up Wide	4 x 2
Pull-up Reverse	4 x 2
Pull-up Close	4 x 2
Cliffhangers	4 x 2
Dips	5 x 2

Cardio

Treadmill: Running (miles)	2
or	
Swimming (miles)	0.75

Other

Rope Climb	30 feet x 1
Eight Count Body Builder	15

LEVEL 4

Warmup	
Running	1.5 miles

Stretch	
Hurdler	L/R 30 sec
or	
Modified Hurdler	L/R 30 sec
Sitting Head to Knee	30 sec
Back Rollers (optional)	30 sec
Butterfly	30 sec
Groin Stretch	30 sec
ITB Stretch	L/R 30 sec
Swimmer Stretch	30 sec
Triceps Stretch	L/R 15 sec
Press-Press-Fling	10
Up Back and Over	10
Trunk Rotations	4
Trunk Benders	5

Upper Body	
Pushup Regular	20 x 2
Pushup Triceps	10 x 2
Pushup Dive Bomber	15 x 2
Arm Haulers	25

Abdominals	
Situp	35 x 2
Leg Lever	35 x 2
Atomic Situp	15 x 2
Back Flutter Kick	30 x 2
Crunches Heel in Close	30 x 2
Crunches Extended Leg	30 x 2
Cross Leg Situp	L/R 18 x 2
Sitting Flutter Kick	15 x 2
Sitting Knee Benders	15 x 2
Scissors	30 x 2
Sitting Bicycles	30 x 2
Neck Rotations	L/R 15 U/D 20

These exercises are optional or substitutes

LEVEL 4

Lower Body

Lunges	25
Squat Leaps	20
Side Lunge	15
Star Jumpers	10

Pull-ups

Pull-up Regular	5 x 2
Pull-up Wide	5 x 2
Pull-up Reverse	5 x 2
Pull-up Close	5 x 2
Cliffhangers	5 x 2
Dips	10 x 3

Cardio

Treadmill: Running (miles)	3
or	
Swimming (miles)	1

Other

Rope Climb	30 feet x 2
Eight Count Body Builder	20

LEVEL 5

Warmup	
Running	2 miles

Stretch	
Hurdler	L/R 30 sec
or	
Modified Hurdler	L/R 30 sec
Sitting Head to Knee	30 sec
Back Rollers (optional)	30 sec
Butterfly	30 sec
Groin Stretch	30 sec
ITB Stretch	L/R 30 sec
Swimmer Stretch	30 sec
Triceps Stretch	L/R 15 sec
Press-Press-Fling	10
Up Back and Over	10
Trunk Rotations	4
Trunk Benders	5

Upper Body	
Pushup Regular	20 x 3
Pushup Triceps	10 x 3
Pushup Dive Bomber	15 x 3
Arm Haulers	30

Abdominals	
Situp	50 x 2
Leg Lever	50 x 2
Atomic Situp	20 x 2
Back Flutter Kick	40 x 2
Crunches Heel in Close	40 x 2
Crunches Extended Leg	40 x 2
Cross Leg Situp	L/R 25 x 2
Sitting Flutter Kick	20 x 2
Sitting Knee Benders	20 x 2
Scissors	40 x 2
Sitting Bicycles	40 x 2
Neck Rotations	L/R 15 U/D 20

These exercises are optional or substitutes

LEVEL 5

Lower Body

Lunges	30
Squat Leaps	25
Side Lunge	20
Star Jumpers	15

Pull-ups

Pull-up Regular	6 x 2
Pull-up Wide	6 x 2
Pull-up Reverse	6 x 2
Pull-up Close	6 x 2
Cliffhangers	6 x 2
Dips	15 x 3

Cardio

Treadmill: Running (miles)	4
or	
Swimming (miles)	1.5

Other

Rope Climb	30 feet x 3
Eight Count Body Builder	25

A BRIEF HISTORY OF THE BATES 924:
THE OFFICIAL TRAINING BOOT OF THE US NAVY SEALS

Note: Many people have asked, "What kind of boots do the Navy SEALs wear? How can anyone run five miles in boots?"

This section will provide some interesting insight into the history and performance of the training boot worn by the Navy SEALs. I appreciate the help of Andrea Poe and Keith Anderson of Bates Uniform Footwear for their assistance in preparing this chapter.

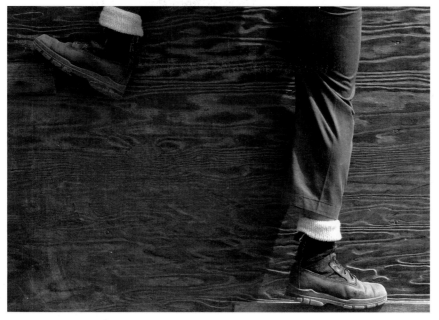

A MISSION

The Bates Shoe Company earned its reputation the right way. It has crafted the highest quality uniform footwear since 1885, and its commitment has not wavered since that time. The 924 is the latest example of the success that can be achieved, with a focus on precision, on performance, and on quality. Now Bates footwear serves more than 50 of the world's military forces and countless civil servants and law enforcement agencies around the globe. Its mission is to provide high-tech performance gear that is an integral part of the equipment put into action by military and law enforcement personnel everyday. And the gear speaks for itself: The Bates brand stands for performance and precision to both military and civilian forces.

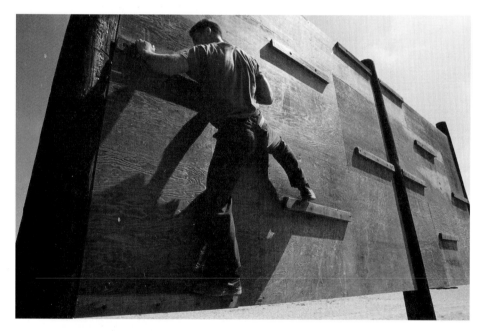

Hangin' out on the Spider Wall, Navy SEAL O' Course.

A CALL TO ACTION

The Bates brand dominates the global market for uniform footwear. The company achieved this position by listening and by responding to the military's critical footwear needs. Bates managers visit training facilities and military academic institutions throughout the year to receive product feedback from their users, and with this information they make continuous improvements to existing products, fueling ideas for innovative new designs.

In 1993, Bates responded to the military's need for a lighter, more comfortable training shoe. The boot designed to serve this need is now widely known as the Bates 924.

EXCELLENCE BY DESIGN

There are several reasons the Bates 924 and 918 steel toe version outperform other training boots. The 924's major features are the Durashocks® Comfort System, leather/cordura uppers, Direct Attach construction and a unique slip resistant sole. These features combine to offer the world's most comfortable military boot.

The DuraShocks® Comfort System

The DuraShocks® Comfort System absorbs shock with compression pads in the heel and forepart of the DuraShocks® outsole. Axidyne® Polymer—the same cushioning used inside football helmets—is used to help to return energy to the foot as the heel lifts after impact. The Durashocks® outsole itself is as flexible as a running shoe.

The DuraShocks® construction is lightweight. Polyurethane compounds used in the 924 outsole weigh one fourth as much as standard rubber sole compounds, yet absorb and return several times the energy. This results in less fatigue and less wasted energy exerted by the wearer.

Lightweight Leather and Cordura® Uppers

The combination of leather and Cordura® in the 924 uppers allows a lightweight toughness and exceptional wear performance. Cordura® was chosen for its exceptional resistance to abrasions, punctures and tear and for its resistance to mildew. Together, these materials give the 924 strength to wear well and dependably, while maintaining an attractive appearance.

Direct Attach Construction

Direct Attach construction was pioneered by Bates for its superior shock absorbing qualities compared to the standard welt issue construction, and for its waterproofing capabilities.

In the final analysis, Direct Attach design offers a superior level of shock absorption at heel strike and is more efficient in returning energy to the wearer. In fact, the shock absorption quality of the boot is comparable to running shoes like the Nike® Air Max. Evidence of the 924's performance ability comes straight from the Biomechanical Research Labs at Michigan State University, where the boot was tested under highly controlled conditions. Because of Direct Attach construction, the 924 is also superior in terms of fore foot flexibility, an important factor in reducing foot fatigue and injury.

A Flexible, Slip Resistant Outsole

The 924's slip resistant polyurethane outsole provides a flexible base for action. This unique dual density outsole remains flexible over the life of the shoe because of its unique cellular makeup—and a manufacturing process that insures the finished material will not break down under heavy use. Polyurethane soles and heels also act as an insulator, keeping feet cooler in the summer and warmer in the winter.

ULTIMATE LEADERSHIP

Bates currently has upwards of 50 percent market share in the uni-form footwear industry and today, Bates Style No. 924 is the proud official training boot of the U.S. Navy SEALs. The Bates 924 is not a standard issue boot, although it can be purchased through Military and Navy exchanges throughout the US. Bates footwear continues to be the major supplier of the Naval Academy, Air Force Academy, West Point, and the Merchant Marine Academy.

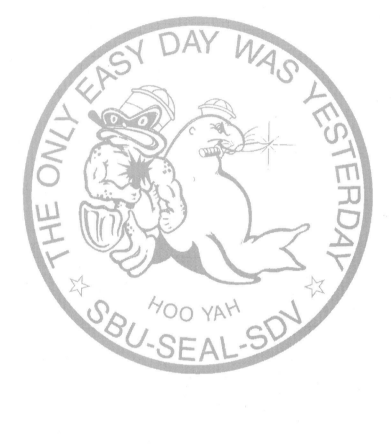

NAVY SEAL RECRUITING INFORMATION

FOR MORE INFORMATION ABOUT BECOMING A NAVY SEAL, SPEAK WITH YOUR LOCAL NAVY RECRUITER OR CONTACT:

SEAL Recruiter
Naval Special Warfare
2446 Trident Way
San Diego, CA 92155-5494
Com. (619) 437-3641/3656
DSN 577-3641

SEAL Detailer
Bureau of Naval Personnel
Pers 401D
Navy Annex
Washington, D. C. 20370
(703) 614-1091

Officer Detailer
Bureau of Naval Personnel
Pers 415
2 Navy Annex
Washington, D. C. 20370
(703) 614-8327

Dive Motivators (SEAL)
Bldg. 1405
Recruit Training Command
Great Lakes, IL 60088
(708) 688-4643

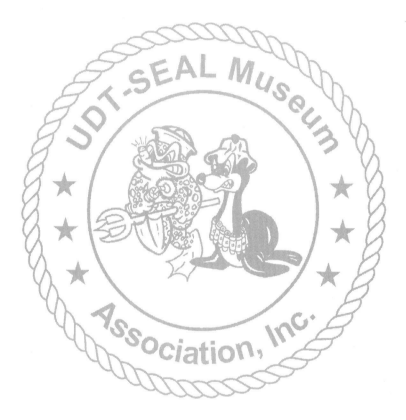

UDT-SEAL MUSEUM ASSOCIATION, INC.

The Underwater Demolition Teams—better known as Frogmen—and the SEAL Teams, along with the Scouts & Raiders and the Naval Combat Demolition Units, have a history shrouded in secrecy. The SEALs are one of our country's most highly decorated combat units. They have earned three Medals of Honor, as well as numerous Navy Crosses, Legions of Merit, Silver Stars, and hundreds of other medals.

The UDT-SEAL Museum is the only museum in the world dedicated exclusively to these elite fighting men.

The UDT-SEAL Museum is located on the original training ground of the U.S. Navy Frogmen in Fort Pierce, Florida. These unique underwater warriors were born here in May 1943.

Now's the time to join the UDT-SEAL Museum Association!

Help preserve the heritage of the Underwater Demolition Teams and the SEAL Teams of the U.S. Navy! Begin/renew membership, volunteer for the Association, and give a gift membership.

For more information on the UDT-SEAL Museum, write, call, or visit:

UDT-SEAL MUSEUM

3300 North A1A • North Hutchinson Island
Fort Pierce, FL 34949-8520 • Phone (561) 595-5845

Hours: Tuesday - Saturday, 10:00 a.m. - 4:00 p.m.
Sunday, Noon - 4:00 p.m.
Open Monday, January 1 - May 1
Adults $3.25 • Children 6 - 12 $1.50 • Pre-Schoolers Free

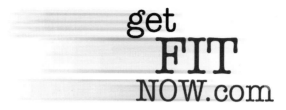

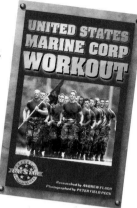

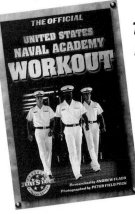

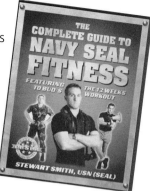

The Navy SEALs Workout Video

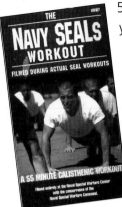

55 minutes of the most intense total body workout you've ever seen!

Filmed during actual SEAL workouts, this calisthenics workout is guaranteed to get you into "fighting shape" the SEAL way—by the same proven program that produces these special men trained to prevail from sea, land, or air.

The physical training is led on-camera by veteran SEAL instructors who demonstrate proper techniques and instill the special spirit and motivation to succeed for which the SEALs are renowned.

Come participate in the physical training of the most versatile, best-conditioned military unit in the world with **The Navy SEALs Workout!**

Check out this and other exciting fitness books, video, and equipment at our website: www.getfitnow.com

Just $19.95
plus $3.00 S/H

To order call toll-free 1-800-906-1234

VISA • MASTERCARD • AMERICAN EXPRESS • DISCOVER
CHECK OR MONEY ORDER TO:
The Hatherleigh Company, Ltd.
1114 First Ave., Suite 500, Dept SS
New York, NY 10021

ABOUT THE AUTHORS

ANDREW FLACH

A lifelong fitness enthusiast, Andrew was born and raised in New York City, and is a graduate of St. David's School, The Browning School, and Vassar College. When he is not running a multi-million dollar media business, his recreational pursuits include sailing, mountaineering, rock climbing, mountain biking, SCUBA diving, and flying. He still resides in New York City.

PETER FIELD PECK

Peter Field Peck is a freelance photographer. His work has appeared in newspapers, magazines, and books. He currently resides in Brattleboro, Vermont.